INDIAN COOKBOOK 2022

TRADITIONAL AND ORIGINAL INDIAN RECIPES

TALA WRIGHT

Table of Contents

Garlic Raita 18
    Ingredients 18
    Method 18
Mixed Vegetable Raita 19
    Ingredients 19
    Method 19
Boondi Raita 20
    Ingredients 20
    Method 20
Cauliflower Raita 21
    Ingredients 21
    Method 22
Cabbage Raita 23
    Ingredients 23
    Method 23
Beetroot Raita 24
    Ingredients 24
    Method 24
Sprouted Pulses Raita 25
    Ingredients 25
    Method 25
Pasta Pudina Raita 26
    Ingredients 26

- Method 26
- Mint Raita 27
  - Ingredients 27
  - Method 27
- Aubergine Raita 28
  - Ingredients 28
  - Method 28
- Saffron Raita 29
  - Ingredients 29
  - Method 29
- Yam Raita 30
  - Ingredients 30
  - Method 31
- Okra Raita 32
  - Ingredients 32
  - Method 32
- Crunchy Spinach Patty 33
  - Ingredients 33
  - Method 33
- Rava Dosa 35
  - Ingredients 35
  - Method 35
- Doodhi Cutlet 36
  - Ingredients 36
  - For the white sauce: 36
  - Method 36
- Patra 38

Ingredients	38
For the batter:	38
Method	39
Nargisi Chicken Kebab	**40**
Ingredients	40
Method	41
Sev Puris with Savoury Topping	**42**
Ingredients	42
Method	43
Special Roll	**44**
Ingredients	44
Method	45
Fried Colocasia	**46**
Ingredients	46
Method	47
Mixed Dhal Dosa	**48**
Ingredients	48
Method	48
Makkai Cakes	**49**
Ingredients	49
Method	50
Hara Bhara Kebab	**51**
Ingredients	51
Method	51
Fish Pakoda	**53**
Ingredients	53
Method	54

- Shammi Kebab 55
  - Ingredients 55
  - Method 56
- Basic Dhokla 57
  - Ingredients 57
  - Method 58
- Adai 59
  - Ingredients 59
  - Method 60
- Double Decker Dhokla 61
  - Ingredients 61
  - Method 62
- Ulundu Vada 63
  - Ingredients 63
  - Method 63
- Bhakar Wadi 64
  - Ingredients 64
  - Method 64
- Mangalorean Chaat 66
  - Ingredients 66
  - Method 67
- Pani Puri 68
  - Ingredients 68
  - For the stuffing: 68
  - For the pani: 68
  - Method 69
- Stuffed Spinach Egg 70

Ingredients	70
Method	71
Sada Dosa	72
Ingredients	72
Method	72
Potato Samosa	74
Ingredients	74
Method	75
Hot Kachori	76
Ingredients	76
Method	76
Khandvi	78
Ingredients	78
Method	79
Makkai Squares	80
Ingredients	80
Method	81
Dhal Pakwan	82
Ingredients	82
For the pakwan:	82
Method	83
Spicy Sev	84
Ingredients	84
Method	84
Stuffed Veggie Crescents	85
Ingredients	85
For the filling:	85

- Method 86
- Kachori Usal 87
  - Ingredients 87
  - For the filling: 87
  - For the sauce: 88
  - Method 88
- Dhal Dhokli 90
  - Ingredients 90
  - For the dhal: 90
  - Method 91
- Misal 92
  - Ingredients 92
  - For the spice mixture: 93
  - Method 94
- Pandori 95
  - Ingredients 95
  - Method 95
- Vegetable Adai 96
  - Ingredients 96
  - Method 97
- Spicy Corn on the Cob 98
  - Ingredients 98
  - Method 98
- Mixed Vegetable Chop 99
  - Ingredients 99
  - Method 100
- Idli Upma 101

- Ingredients 101
  - Method 102
- Dhal Bhajiya 103
  - Ingredients 103
  - Method 103
- Masala Papad 104
  - Ingredients 104
  - Method 104
- Vegetable Sandwich 105
  - Ingredients 105
  - Method 105
- Sprouted Mung Bean Rolls 106
  - Ingredients 106
  - Method 107
- Chutney Sandwich 108
  - Ingredients 108
  - Method 108
- Chatpata Gobhi 109
  - Ingredients 109
  - Method 109
- Sabudana Vada 110
  - Ingredients 110
  - Method 110
- Bread Upma 111
  - Ingredients 111
  - Method 112
- Spicy Khaja 113

- Ingredients 113
  - Method 114
- Crispy Potato 115
  - Ingredients 115
  - Method 116
- Dhal Vada 117
  - Ingredients 117
  - Method 118
- Zunka 119
  - Ingredients 119
  - Method 119
- Turnip Curry 121
  - Ingredients 121
  - Method 122
- Chhaner Dhalna 123
  - Ingredients 123
  - Method 124
- Corn with Coconut 125
  - Ingredients 125
  - For the coconut paste: 125
  - Method 126
- Green Pepper with Potato 127
  - Ingredients 127
  - Method 128
- Spicy Peas with Potatoes 129
  - Ingredients 129
  - Method 130

- Sautéed Mushrooms 131
  - Ingredients 131
  - Method 131
- Spicy Mushroom with Baby Corn 132
  - Ingredients 132
  - Method 133
- Dry Spicy Cauliflower 134
  - Ingredients 134
  - Method 135
- Mushroom Curry 136
  - Ingredients 136
  - Method 137
- Baingan Bharta 138
  - Ingredients 138
  - Method 139
- Vegetable Hyderabadi 140
  - Ingredients 140
  - For the spice mixture: 140
  - Method 141
- Kaddu Bhaji* 142
  - Ingredients 142
  - Method 143
- Muthia nu Shak 144
  - Ingredients 144
  - Method 145
- Pumpkin Koot 146
  - Ingredients 146

Method	147
Rassa	148
Ingredients	148
Method	149
Doodhi Manpasand	150
Ingredients	150
Method	151
Tomato Chokha	152
Ingredients	152
Method	152
Baingan Chokha	153
Ingredients	153
Method	153
Cauliflower & Peas Curry	154
Ingredients	154
Method	154
Aloo Methi ki Sabzi	155
Ingredients	155
Method	155
Sweet & Sour Karela	156
Ingredients	156
Method	157
Karela Koshimbir	158
Ingredients	158
Method	158
Karela Curry	159
Ingredients	159

- Method 160
- Chilli Cauliflower 161
  - Ingredients 161
  - Method 161
- Nutty Curry 162
  - Ingredients 162
  - Method 163
- Daikon Leaves Bhaaji 164
  - Ingredients 164
  - Method 164
- Chhole Aloo 165
  - Ingredients 165
  - Method 166
- Peanut Curry 167
  - Ingredients 167
  - Method 168
- French Beans Upkari 169
  - Ingredients 169
  - Method 169
- Karatey Ambadey 170
  - Ingredients 170
  - Method 171
- Kadhai Paneer 172
  - Ingredients 172
  - Method 172
- Kathirikkai Vangi 173
  - Ingredients 173

- Method 174
- Pitla 175
  - Ingredients 175
  - Method 176
- Cauliflower Masala 177
  - Ingredients 177
  - For the sauce: 177
  - Method 178
- Shukna Kacha Pepe 179
  - Ingredients 179
  - Method 180
- Dry Okra 181
  - Ingredients 181
  - Method 181
- Moghlai Cauliflower 182
  - Ingredients 182
  - Method 182
- Bhapa Shorshe Baingan 183
  - Ingredients 183
  - Method 184
- Baked Vegetables in Spicy Sauce 185
  - Ingredients 185
  - Method 186
- Tasty Tofu 187
  - Ingredients 187
  - Method 187
- Aloo Baingan 188

- Ingredients 188
  - Method 189
- Sugar Snap Pea Curry 190
  - Ingredients 190
  - Method 190
- Potato Pumpkin Curry 191
  - Ingredients 191
  - Method 192
- Egg Thoran 193
  - Ingredients 193
  - Method 194
- Baingan Lajawab 195
  - Ingredients 195
  - Method 196
- Veggie Bahar 197
  - Ingredients 197
  - Method 198
- Stuffed Vegetables 199
  - Ingredients 199
  - For the filling: 199
  - Method 200
- Singhi Aloo 201
  - Ingredients 201
  - Method 201
- Sindhi Curry 202
  - Ingredients 202
  - Method 203

Gulnar Kofta 204
    Ingredients 204
    For the spice mixture: 204
    Method 205
Paneer Korma 206
    Ingredients 206
    Method 207
Chutney Potatoes 208
    Ingredients 208
    Method 209
Lobia 210
    Ingredients 210
    Method 211
Khatta Meetha Vegetable 212
    Ingredients 212
    Method 213
Dahiwale Chhole 214
    Ingredients 214
    Method 215
Teekha Papad Bhaji* 216
    Ingredients 216
    Method 216

Garlic Raita

Serves 4

Ingredients

2 green chillies

5 garlic cloves

450g/1lb yoghurt, whisked

Salt to taste

Method

- Dry roast the chillies till they turn light brown. Grind them with the garlic.
- Mix with the remaining ingredients. Serve chilled.

Mixed Vegetable Raita

Serves 4

Ingredients

1 large potato, finely diced and boiled

25g/scant 1oz French beans, finely diced and boiled

25g/scant 1oz carrots, finely diced and boiled

50g/1¾oz boiled peas

450g/1lb yoghurt

½ tsp ground black pepper

1 tbsp coriander leaves, finely chopped

Salt to taste

Method

- Mix all the ingredients well in a bowl. Serve chilled.

Boondi Raita

Serves 4

Ingredients

115g/4oz salted boondi*

450g/1lb yoghurt

½ tsp sugar

½ tsp chaat masala*

Method

- Mix all the ingredients well in a bowl. Serve chilled.

Cauliflower Raita

Serves 4

Ingredients

250g/9oz cauliflower, chopped into tiny florets, or grated

Salt to taste

½ tsp ground black pepper

½ tsp chilli powder

½ tsp ground mustard

450g/1lb yoghurt

1 tsp ghee

½ tsp mustard seeds

Chaat masala* to taste

Method

- Mix the cauliflower with salt and steam mixture.
- Whisk the pepper, chilli powder, mustard, salt and yoghurt in a bowl.
- Add the cauliflower mixture to the yoghurt mixture and set aside.
- Heat the ghee in a small saucepan. When it begins to smoke, add the mustard seeds. Let them splutter for 15 seconds.
- Add this with the chaat masala to the yoghurt mixture. Serve chilled.

Cabbage Raita

Serves 4

Ingredients

100g/3½oz cabbage, grated

Salt to taste

1 tbsp coriander leaves, finely chopped

2 tsp grated coconut

450g/1lb yoghurt

1 tsp oil

½ tsp mustard seeds

3-4 curry leaves

Method

- Steam the cabbage with salt. Let it cool down.
- Add the coriander leaves, coconut and yoghurt. Mix well. Set aside.
- Heat the oil in a small saucepan. Add the mustard seeds and curry leaves. Let them splutter for 15 seconds.
- Pour this in the yoghurt mixture. Serve chilled.

Beetroot Raita

Serves 4

Ingredients

1 large beetroot, boiled and grated

450g/1lb yoghurt

½ tsp sugar

Salt to taste

1 tsp ghee

½ tsp cumin seeds

1 green chilli, slit lengthways

1 tbsp coriander leaves, finely chopped

Method

- Mix the beetroot, yoghurt, sugar and salt in a bowl.
- Heat the ghee in a saucepan. Add the cumin seeds and green chilli. Let them splutter for 15 seconds. Add this to the beetroot-yoghurt mixture.
- Transfer to a serving bowl and garnish with the coriander leaves.
- Serve chilled.

Sprouted Pulses Raita

Serves 4

Ingredients

75g/2½oz bean sprouts

75g/2½oz sprouted kaala chana*

75g/2½oz sprouted chickpeas

1 cucumber, finely chopped

10g/¼oz coriander leaves, finely chopped

2 tsp chaat masala*

½ tsp sugar

450g/1lb yoghurt

Method

- Steam the bean sprouts for 5 minutes. Set aside.
- Boil the kaala chana and chickpeas along with some water on a medium heat in a saucepan for 30 minutes. Set aside.
- Mix the bean sprouts with all the remaining ingredients. Mix well. Drain and add the kaala chana and chickpeas.
- Serve chilled.

Pasta Pudina Raita

Serves 4

Ingredients

200g/7oz pasta, boiled

1 large cucumber, finely chopped

450g/1lb yoghurt, whisked

2 tsp ready-made mustard

50g/1¾oz mint leaves, finely chopped

Salt to taste

Method

- Mix all the ingredients together. Serve chilled.

Mint Raita

Serves 4

Ingredients

50g/1¾oz mint leaves

25g/scant 1oz coriander leaves

1 green chilli

2 garlic cloves

450g/1lb yoghurt

1 tsp chaat masala*

1 tsp caster sugar

Salt to taste

Method

- Grind together the mint leaves, coriander leaves, green chilli and garlic.
- Mix with the other ingredients in a bowl.
- Serve chilled.

Aubergine Raita

Serves 4

Ingredients

1 large aubergine

450g/1lb yoghurt

1 large onion, finely grated

2 green chillies, finely chopped

10g/¼oz coriander leaves, finely chopped

Salt to taste

Method

- Pierce the aubergine all over with a fork. Roast in the oven at 180ºC (350ºF, Gas Mark 4) turning it occasionally, till the skin is charred.
- Soak the aubergine in a bowl of water to cool it down. Drain the water and peel off the aubergine skin.
- Mash the aubergine till smooth. Mix with all the other ingredients.
- Serve chilled.

Saffron Raita

Serves 4

Ingredients

350g/12oz yoghurt

1 tsp saffron, soaked in 2 tbsp milk for 30 minutes

25g/scant 1oz raisins, soaked in water for 2 hours

75g/2½oz roasted almonds and pistachios, finely chopped

1 tbsp caster sugar

Method

- In a bowl, whisk the yoghurt with the saffron.
- Add all the other ingredients. Mix well.
- Serve chilled.

Yam Raita

Serves 4

Ingredients

250g/9oz yams*

Salt to taste

¼ tsp chilli powder

¼ tsp ground black pepper

350g/12oz yoghurt

1 tsp ghee

½ tsp cumin seeds

2 green chillies, slit lengthways

1 tbsp coriander leaves, finely chopped

Method

- Peel and grate the yams. Add some salt and steam the mixture till soft. Set aside.
- In a bowl, mix the salt, chilli powder and ground pepper with the yoghurt.
- Add the yam to the yoghurt mixture. Set aside.
- Heat the ghee in a small saucepan. Add the cumin seeds and green chillies. Let them splutter for 15 seconds.
- Add this to the yoghurt mixture. Mix gently.
- Garnish with the coriander leaves. Serve chilled.

Okra Raita

Serves 4

Ingredients

250g/9oz okra, finely chopped

Salt to taste

½ tsp chilli powder

½ tsp turmeric

Refined vegetable oil for deep frying

350g/12oz yoghurt

1 tsp chaat masala*

Method

- Rub the okra pieces with the salt, chilli powder and turmeric.
- Heat the oil in a saucepan. Deep fry the okra on a medium heat for 3-4 minutes. Drain on absorbent paper. Set aside.
- In a bowl, whisk the yoghurt with the chaat masala and salt.
- Add the fried okra to the yoghurt mixture.
- Serve chilled or at room temperature.

Crunchy Spinach Patty

Makes 12

Ingredients

1 tbsp refined vegetable oil plus extra for deep frying

1 large onion, finely chopped

50g/1¾oz spinach, boiled and finely chopped

1 tsp garlic paste

1 tsp ginger paste

Salt to taste

300g/10oz paneer*, chopped

2 eggs, whisked

2 tbsp plain white flour

Pepper to taste

Salt to taste

50g/1¾oz breadcrumbs

Method

- Heat the oil in a frying pan. Fry the onion on a medium heat till translucent.
- Add the spinach, garlic paste, ginger paste and salt. Cook for 2-3 minutes.

- Remove from the heat and add the paneer. Mix well and divide into square patties. Cover with foil and refrigerate for 30 minutes.
- Mix the eggs, flour, pepper and salt together to form a smooth batter.
- Heat the remaining oil in a frying pan. Dip each paneer patty into the batter, roll in the breadcrumbs and deep fry till golden brown.
- Serve hot with dry garlic chutney

Rava Dosa

(Semolina Crêpe)

Makes 10-12

Ingredients

100g/3½oz semolina

85g/3oz plain white flour

Pinch of bicarbonate of soda

250g/9oz yoghurt

240ml/8fl oz water

Salt to taste

Refined vegetable oil for greasing

Method

- Blend all the ingredients, except the oil, together to form a batter of a pancake-mix consistency. Set aside for 20-30 minutes.
- Grease and heat a flat pan. Pour 2 tbsp of batter in it. Spread by lifting the pan and rotating it gently.
- Pour some oil around the edges.
- Cook for 3 minutes. Flip and cook till crisp.
- Repeat for the remaining batter.
- Serve hot with coconut chutney

Doodhi Cutlet

(Bottle Gourd Cutlet)

Makes 20

Ingredients

1 tbsp refined vegetable oil plus extra for frying

1 large onion, chopped

4 green chillies, finely chopped

2.5cm/1in root ginger, grated

1 large bottle gourd*, peeled and grated

Salt to taste

2 eggs, whisked

100g/3½oz breadcrumbs

For the white sauce:

2 tbsp margarine/butter

4 tbsp flour

Salt to taste

Pepper to taste

1 tbsp cream

Method

- For the white sauce, heat the margarine/butter in a saucepan.
  Add all the remaining white sauce ingredients and stir on a medium heat till thick and creamy. Set aside.
- Heat the oil in a frying pan. Fry the onion, green chillies and ginger on a medium heat for 2-3 minutes.
- Add the bottle gourd and salt. Mix well. Cover with a lid and cook for 15-20 minutes on a medium heat.
- Uncover and mash the bottle gourd well. Add the white sauce and half the whisked eggs. Set aside for 20 minutes to harden and set.
- Chop the mixture into cutlets.
- Heat the oil in a saucepan. Dip each cutlet in the remaining whisked egg, roll in the breadcrumbs and deep fry till golden brown.
- Serve hot with sweet tomato chutney

Patra

(Colocasia Leaf Pinwheel)

Makes 20

Ingredients

10 colocasia leaves*

2 tbsp refined vegetable oil

½ tsp mustard seeds

1 tsp sesame seeds

1 tsp cumin seeds

8 curry leaves

2 tbsp coriander leaves, finely chopped

For the batter:

250g/9oz besan*

4 tbsp jaggery*, grated

1 tsp tamarind paste

½ tsp ginger paste

½ tsp garlic paste

1 tsp chilli powder

½ tsp turmeric

Salt to taste

Method

- Mix all the batter ingredients to form a thick batter.
- Spread a layer of the batter on each colocasia leaf to cover it completely.
- Place 5 coated leaves one above the other.
- Fold the leaves 2.5cm/1in from each corner to form a square. Roll this square into a cylinder.
- Repeat for the other 5 leaves.
- Steam the rolls for about 20-25 minutes. Set aside to cool.
- Slice each roll into pinwheel-like shapes. Set aside.
- Heat the oil in a saucepan. Add the mustard, sesame seeds, cumin seeds and curry leaves. Let them splutter for 15 seconds.
- Pour this over the pinwheels.
- Garnish with the coriander leaves. Serve hot.

Nargisi Chicken Kebab

(Chicken and Cheese Kebab)

Makes 20-25

Ingredients

500g/1lb 2oz chicken, minced

150g/5½oz grated Cheddar cheese

2 large onions, finely chopped

1 tsp ginger paste

1 tsp garlic paste

1 tsp ground cardamom

2 tsp garam masala

1 tsp ground coriander

½ tsp turmeric

½ tsp chilli powder

Salt to taste

15-20 raisins

Refined vegetable oil for deep frying

Method

- Knead all the ingredients, except the raisins and oil, into a dough.
- Make small dumplings. Place a raisin in the centre of each dumpling.
- Heat the oil in a frying pan. Fry the dumplings on a medium heat till golden brown. Serve hot with mint chutney

Sev Puris with Savoury Topping

Serves 4

Ingredients

24 sev puris*

2 potatoes, diced and boiled

1 large onion, finely chopped

¼ small unripe green mango, finely chopped

120ml/4fl oz hot and sour chutney

4 tbsp mint chutney

1 tsp chaat masala*

Juice of 1 lemon

Salt to taste

150g/5½oz sev*

2 tbsp coriander leaves, chopped

Method

- Arrange the puris on a serving plate.
- Place small portions of the potatoes, onion and mango on each puri.
- Sprinkle the hot and sour chutney and mint chutney on top of each puri.
- Sprinkle the chaat masala, lemon juice and salt on top.
- Garnish with the sev and coriander leaves. Serve immediately.

Special Roll

Makes 4

Ingredients

1 tsp yeast

Pinch of sugar

240ml/8fl oz warm water

350g/12oz plain white flour

½ tsp baking powder

2 tbsp butter

1 large onion, finely chopped

2 tomatoes, finely chopped

30g/1oz mint leaves, finely chopped

200g/7oz spinach, boiled

300g/10oz paneer*, diced

Salt to taste

Ground black pepper to taste

125g/4½oz tomato purée

1 egg, whisked

Method

- Dissolve the yeast and sugar in the water.
- Sieve the flour and baking powder together. Mix with the yeast and knead into a dough.
- With a rolling pin, roll out the dough into 2 chapattis. Set aside.
- Heat half the butter in a saucepan. Add the onion, tomatoes, mint leaves, spinach, paneer, salt and black pepper. Sauté on a medium heat for 3 minutes.
- Spread this over 1 chapatti. Pour the tomato purée on top and cover with the other chapatti. Seal the ends.
- Brush the chapattis with the egg and remaining butter.
- Bake in an oven at 150ºC (300ºF, Gas Mark 2) for 10 minutes. Serve hot.

Fried Colocasia

Serves 4

Ingredients

500g/1lb 2 oz colocasia*

2 tbsp ground coriander

1 tbsp ground cumin

1 tbsp amchoor*

2 tsp besan*

Salt to taste

Refined vegetable oil for frying

Chaat masala*, to taste

1 tbsp coriander leaves, chopped

½ tsp lemon juice

Method

- Boil the colocasia in a saucepan for 15 minutes on a low heat. Cool, peel, cut lengthways and flatten. Set aside.
- Mix the ground coriander, ground cumin, amchoor, besan and salt. Roll the colocasia pieces in this mixture. Set aside.
- Heat the oil in a saucepan. Deep fry the colocasia till crisp, then drain.
- Sprinkle with the remaining ingredients. Serve hot.

Mixed Dhal Dosa

(Mixed Lentil Crêpe)

Makes 8-10

Ingredients

250g/9oz rice, soaked for 5-6 hours

100g/3½oz mung dhal*, soaked for 5-6 hours

100g/3½oz chana dhal*, soaked for 5-6 hours

100g/3½oz urad dhal*, soaked for 5-6 hours

2 tbsp yoghurt

½ tsp bicarbonate of soda

2 tbsp refined vegetable oil plus extra for frying

Salt to taste

Method

- Wet grind the rice and the dhals separately. Mix together. Add the yoghurt, bicarbonate of soda, oil and salt. Whisk till fluffy and light. Set aside for 3-4 hours.
- Grease and heat a flat pan. Pour 2 tbsp of batter over it and spread like a crêpe. Pour some oil around the edges. Cook for 2 minutes. Serve hot.

Makkai Cakes

(Corn Cakes)

Makes 12-15

Ingredients

4 fresh corn cobs

2 tbsp butter

750ml/1¼ pints milk

½ tsp chilli powder

Salt to taste

Ground black pepper to taste

25g/scant 1oz coriander leaves, chopped

50g/1¾oz breadcrumbs

Method

- Remove the kernels from the corn cobs and grind them coarsely.
- Heat the butter in a saucepan and fry the ground corn for 2-3 minutes on a medium heat. Add the milk and simmer till dry.
- Add the chilli powder, salt, black pepper and coriander leaves.
- Add the breadcrumbs and mix well. Divide the mixture into small patties.
- Heat the butter in a frying pan. Shallow fry the patties till golden brown. Serve hot with ketchup.

Hara Bhara Kebab

(Green Vegetable Kebab)

Serves 4

Ingredients

300g/10oz chana dhal*, soaked overnight

2 green cardamom pods

2.5cm/1in cinnamon

Salt to taste

60ml/2fl oz water

200g/7oz spinach, steamed and ground

½ tsp garam masala

¼ tsp mace, grated

Refined vegetable oil to shallow fry

Method

- Drain the dhal. Add the cardamom, cloves, cinnamon, salt and water. Cook in a saucepan on a medium heat till soft. Grind to a paste.
- Add all the remaining ingredients, except the oil. Mix well. Divide the mixture into lemon-sized balls and flatten each into small patties.

- Heat the oil in a frying pan. Shallow fry the patties over a medium heat till golden brown. Serve hot with mint chutney

Fish Pakoda

(Battered Fried Fish)

Makes 12

Ingredients

300g/10oz boneless fish, chopped into 2.5cm/1in pieces

Salt to taste

2 tsp lemon juice

3 tbsp water

250g/9oz besan*

1 tsp garlic paste

2 green chillies, finely chopped

1 tsp garam masala

½ tsp turmeric

Refined vegetable oil for deep frying

Method

- Marinate the fish with the salt and lemon juice for 20 minutes.
- Mix the remaining ingredients, except the oil, to make a thick batter.
- Heat the oil in a saucepan. Dip each piece of fish in the batter and fry till golden. Drain on absorbent paper. Serve hot.

Shammi Kebab

(Mince and Bengal Gram Kebab)

Makes 35

Ingredients

750g/1lb 10oz chicken, minced

600g/1lb 5oz chana dhal*

3 large onions, chopped

1 tsp ginger paste

1 tsp garlic paste

2.5cm/1in cinnamon

4 cloves

2 black cardamom pods

7 peppercorns

1 tsp ground cumin

Salt to taste

450ml/15fl oz water

2 eggs, whisked

Refined vegetable oil for frying

Method

- Mix together all the ingredients, except the eggs and oil. Boil in a saucepan till all the water evaporates. Grind to a thick paste.
- Add the eggs to the paste. Mix well. Divide the mixture into 35 patties.
- Heat the oil in a frying pan. Fry the patties on a low heat till golden.
- Serve hot with mint chutney

Basic Dhokla

(Basic Steamed Cake)

Makes 18-20

Ingredients

250g/9oz rice

450g/1lb chana dhal*

60g/2oz yoghurt

¼ tsp bicarbonate of soda

6 green chillies, chopped

1cm/½in root ginger, grated

¼ tsp ground coriander

¼ tsp ground cumin

½ tsp turmeric

Salt to taste

½ coconut, grated

150g/5½oz coriander leaves, finely chopped

1 tbsp refined vegetable oil

½ tsp mustard seeds

Method

- Soak the rice and dhal together for 6 hours. Grind coarsely.
- Add the yoghurt and bicarbonate of soda. Mix well. Let the paste ferment for 6-8 hours.
- Add the green chillies, ginger, ground coriander, ground cumin, turmeric and salt to the batter. Mix thoroughly.
- Pour into a 20cm/8in round cake tin. Steam the batter for 10 minutes.
- Cool and chop into square pieces. Sprinkle the grated coconut and coriander leaves over them. Set aside.
- Heat the oil in a saucepan. Add the mustard seeds. Let them splutter for 15 seconds.
- Pour this over the dhoklas. Serve hot.

Adai

(Rice and Lentil Crêpe)

Makes 12

Ingredients

125g/4½oz rice

75g/2½oz urad dhal*

75g/2½oz chana dhal*

75g/2½oz masoor dhal*

75g/2½oz mung dhal*

6 red chillies

Salt to taste

240ml/8fl oz water

Refined vegetable oil for greasing

Method

- Soak the rice with all the dhals overnight.
- Drain the mixture and add the red chillies, salt and water. Grind until smooth.
- Grease and heat a flat pan. Spread 3 tbsp of the batter on it. Cover and cook on a medium heat for 2-3 minutes. Flip and cook the other side.
- Remove carefully with a spatula. Repeat for the rest of the batter. Serve hot.

Double Decker Dhokla

(Steamed Double Decker Cake)

Makes 20

Ingredients

500g/1lb 2oz rice

300g/10oz urad beans*

75g/2½oz urad dhal*

75g/2½oz chana dhal*

75g/2½oz masoor dhal*

2 green chillies

500g/1lb 2oz yoghurt

1 tsp chilli powder

½ tsp turmeric

Salt to taste

115g/4oz mint chutney

Method

- Mix the rice and urad beans. Soak overnight.
- Mix all the dhals. Soak overnight.
- Drain and grind the rice mixture and the dhal mixture separately. Set aside.
- Mix the green chillies, yoghurt, chilli powder, turmeric and salt together. Add half of this blend to the rice mixture and add the remaining to the dhal mixture. Allow to ferment for 6 hours.
- Grease a 20cm/8in round cake tin. Pour the rice mixture into it. Sprinkle the mint chutney on top of the rice mixture. Pour the dhal mixture on top.
- Steam for 7-8 minutes. Chop and serve hot.

Ulundu Vada

(Fried Doughnut-shaped Snack)

Makes 12

Ingredients

600g/1lb 5oz urad dhal*, soaked overnight and drained

4 green chillies, finely chopped

Salt to taste

3 tbsp water

Refined vegetable oil for deep frying

Method

- Grind the dhal with the green chillies, salt and water.
- Shape the mixture into doughnuts.
- Heat the oil in a saucepan. Add the vadas and deep fry on a medium heat till brown.
- Drain on absorbent paper. Serve hot with coconut chutney

Bhakar Wadi

(Spicy Gram Flour Pinwheel)

Serves 4

Ingredients

500g/1lb 2oz besan*

175g/6oz wholemeal flour

Salt to taste

Pinch of asafoetida

120ml/4fl oz warm refined vegetable oil plus extra for deep frying

100g/3½oz desiccated coconut

1 tsp sesame seeds

1 tsp poppy seeds

Pinch of sugar

1 tsp chilli powder

25g/scant 1oz coriander leaves, finely chopped

1 tbsp tamarind paste

Method

- Knead the besan, flour, salt, asafoetida, warm oil and enough water into a stiff dough. Set aside.

- Dry roast the coconut, sesame seeds and poppy seeds for 3-5 minutes. Grind to a powder.
- Add the sugar, salt, chilli powder, coriander leaves and tamarind paste to the powder and mix thoroughly to prepare the filling. Set aside.
- Divide the dough into lemon-sized balls. Roll each into a thin disc.
- Spread the filling on each disc so that the filling covers the entire disc. Roll each into a tight cylinder. Seal the edges with a little water.
- Slice the cylinders to get pinwheel-like shapes.
- Heat the oil in a saucepan. Add the pinwheel rolls and fry on a medium heat till crisp.
- Drain on absorbent paper. Store in an airtight container once cooled.

NOTE: These can be stored for a fortnight.

Mangalorean Chaat

Serves 4

Ingredients

75g/2½oz chana dhal*

240ml/8fl oz water

Salt to taste

Large pinch of bicarbonate of soda

2 large potatoes, finely chopped and boiled

350g/12oz fresh yoghurt

2 tbsp caster sugar

4 tbsp refined vegetable oil

1 tbsp dried fenugreek leaves

1 tsp ginger paste

1 tsp garlic paste

2 green chillies

1 tsp ground cumin, dry roasted

1 tsp garam masala

1 tbsp amchoor*

1 tsp turmeric

½ tsp chilli powder

150g/5½oz canned chickpeas

1 large onion, finely chopped

2 tbsp coriander leaves, finely chopped

Method

- Cook the dhal with the water, salt and bicarbonate of soda in a saucepan on a medium heat for 30 minutes. Add more water if the dhal feels too dry. Mix the potatoes with the dhal mixture and set aside.
- Whisk the yoghurt with the sugar. Place in the freezer to chill.
- Heat the oil in a saucepan. Add the fenugreek leaves and fry on a medium heat for 3-4 minutes.
- Add the ginger paste, garlic paste, green chillies, ground cumin, garam masala, amchoor, turmeric and chilli powder. Fry for 2-3 minutes, stirring continuously.
- Add the chickpeas. Sauté for 5 minutes, stirring continuously. Add the dhal mixture and mix well.
- Remove from the heat and spread the mixture on a serving platter.
- Pour the sweet yoghurt on top.
- Sprinkle with the onion and coriander leaves. Serve immediately.

Pani Puri

Makes 30

Ingredients
For the puris:

175g/6oz plain white flour

100g/3½oz semolina

Salt to taste

Refined vegetable oil for deep frying

For the stuffing:

50g/1¾oz sprouted mung beans

150g/5½oz sprouted chickpeas

Salt to taste

2 large potatoes, boiled and mashed

For the pani:

2 tbsp tamarind paste

100g/3½oz coriander leaves, finely chopped

1½ tsp ground cumin, dry roasted

2-4 green chillies, finely chopped

2.5cm/1in root ginger

Rock salt to taste

240ml/8fl oz water

Method

- Knead all the puri ingredients, except the oil, with enough water to form a stiff dough.
- Roll out into small puris of 5cm/2in diameter.
- Heat the oil in a frying pan. Deep fry the puris till light brown. Set aside.
- For the stuffing, parboil the sprouted mung beans and chickpeas with the salt. Mix with the potatoes. Set aside.
- For the pani, grind together all the pani ingredients, except the water.
- Add this mixture to the water. Mix well and set aside.
- To serve, make a hole in each puri and fill it with the stuffing. Pour 3 tbsp of the pani into each and serve immediately.

Stuffed Spinach Egg

Serves 4

Ingredients

200g/7oz spinach

Pinch of bicarbonate of soda

1 tbsp refined vegetable oil

1 tsp cumin seeds

6 garlic cloves, crushed

2 green chillies, ground

Salt to taste

8 hard boiled eggs, halved lengthways

1 tbsp ghee

1 onion, finely chopped

2.5cm/1in root ginger, chopped

Method

- Mix the spinach with the bicarbonate of soda. Steam till tender. Grind and set aside.
- Heat the oil in a saucepan. When it begins to smoke, add the cumin seeds, garlic and green chillies. Stir-fry for a few seconds. Add the steamed spinach and salt.
- Cover with a lid and cook till dry. Set aside.
- Scoop the yolks out from the eggs. Add the egg yolks to the spinach mixture. Mix well.
- Place spoonfuls of the spinach-egg mixture in the hollow egg whites. Set aside.
- Heat the ghee in a small frying pan. Fry the onion and ginger till golden brown.
- Sprinkle this on top of the eggs. Serve hot.

Sada Dosa

(Savoury Rice Crêpe)

Makes 15

Ingredients

100g/3½oz parboiled rice

75g/2½oz urad dhal*

½ tsp fenugreek seeds

½ tsp bicarbonate of soda

Salt to taste

125g/4½oz yoghurt, whipped

60ml/2fl oz refined vegetable oil

Method

- Soak the rice and the dhal together with the fenugreek seeds for 7-8 hours.
- Drain and grind the mixture to a grainy paste.
- Add bicarbonate of soda and salt. Mix well.
- Set aside to ferment for 8-10 hours.
- Add the yoghurt to make the batter. This batter should be thick enough to coat a spoon. Add a little water if needed. Set aside.

- Grease and heat a flat pan. Spread a spoonful of the batter over it to make a thin crêpe. Pour 1 tsp oil on top. Cook until crisp. Repeat for the rest of the batter and serve hot.

Potato Samosa

(Potato Savoury)

Makes 20

Ingredients

175g/6oz plain white flour

Pinch of salt

5 tbsp refined vegetable oil plus extra for deep frying

100ml/3½fl oz water

1cm/½in root ginger, grated

2 green chillies, finely chopped

2 garlic cloves, finely chopped

½ tsp ground coriander

1 large onion, finely chopped

2 large potatoes, boiled and mashed

1 tbsp coriander leaves, finely chopped

1 tbsp lemon juice

½ tsp turmeric

1 tsp chilli powder

½ tsp garam masala

Salt to taste

Method

- Mix the flour with the salt, 2 tbsp oil and water. Knead into a pliable dough.
  Cover with a moist cloth and set aside for 15-20 minutes.
- Knead the dough again. Cover with a moist cloth and set aside.
- For the filling, heat 3 tbsp oil in a frying pan. Add the ginger, green chillies, garlic and ground coriander. Fry for a minute on a medium heat, stirring continuously.
- Add the onion and fry till brown.
- Add the potatoes, coriander leaves, lemon juice, turmeric, chilli powder, garam masala and salt. Mix thoroughly.
- Cook on a low heat for 4 minutes, stirring occasionally. Set aside.
- To make the samosas, divide the dough into 10 balls. Roll out into discs of 12cm/5in diameter. Cut each disc into 2 half-moons.
- Run a moist finger along the diameter of a half-moon. Bring the ends together to make a cone.
- Place a tbsp of the filling in the cone and seal by pressing the edges together. Repeat for all the half-moons.
- Heat the oil in a frying pan. Deep fry the samosas, five at a time, over a low heat till light brown. Drain on absorbent paper.
- Serve hot with mint chutney

Hot Kachori

(Fried Dumpling with Lentil Filling)

Makes 15

Ingredients

250g/9oz plain white flour plus 1 tbsp for the patching

5 tbsp refined vegetable oil plus extra for deep frying

Salt to taste

1.4 litres/2½ pints water plus 1 tbsp for patching

300g/10oz mung dhal*, soaked for 30 minutes

½ tsp ground coriander

½ tsp ground fennel

½ tsp cumin seeds

½ tsp mustard seeds

2-3 pinches of asafoetida

1 tsp garam masala

1 tsp chilli powder

Method

- Mix 250g/9oz flour with 3 tbsp oil, salt and 100ml/3½fl oz of the water. Knead into a soft, pliable dough. Set aside for 30 minutes.
- To make the filling, cook the dhal with the remaining water in a saucepan on a medium heat for 45 minutes. Drain and set aside.
- Heat 2 tbsp oil in a saucepan. When it begins to smoke, add the ground coriander, fennel, cumin seeds, mustard seeds, asafoetida, garam masala, chilli powder and salt. Let them splutter for 30 seconds.
- Add the cooked dhal. Mix well and fry for 2-3 minutes, stirring continuously.
- Cool the dhal mixture and divide into 15 lemon-sized balls. Set aside.
- Mix 1 tbsp flour with 1 tbsp water to make a paste for patching. Set aside.
- Divide the dough into 15 balls. Roll out into discs of 12cm/5in diameter.
- Place 1 ball of the filling in the centre of a disc. Seal like a pouch.
- Flatten slightly by pressing it between the palms. Repeat for the remaining discs.
- Heat the oil in a saucepan until it starts smoking. Deep fry the discs till golden brown on the underside. Flip and repeat.
- If a kachori tears while frying, seal it with the patching paste.
- Drain on absorbent paper. Serve hot with mint chutney

Khandvi

(Besan Roll-Ups)

Makes 10-15

Ingredients

60g/2oz besan*

60g/2oz yoghurt

120ml/4fl oz water

1 tsp turmeric

Salt to taste

5 tbsp refined vegetable oil

1 tbsp fresh coconut, grated

1 tbsp coriander leaves, finely chopped

½ tsp mustard seeds

2 pinches of asafoetida

8 curry leaves

2 green chillies, finely chopped

1 tsp sesame seeds

Method

- Mix the besan, yoghurt, water, turmeric and salt together.
- Heat 4 tbsp oil in a frying pan. Add the besan mixture and cook, stirring continuously to make sure no lumps are formed.
- Cook till the mixture leaves the sides of the pan. Set aside.
- Grease two 15 × 35cm/6 × 14in non-stick baking trays. Pour in the besan mixture and smooth flat with a palette knife. Allow to set for 10 minutes.
- Cut the mixture into 5cm/2in wide strips. Carefully roll up each strip.
- Place the rolls in a serving dish. Sprinkle the grated coconut and coriander leaves on top. Set aside.
- Heat 1 tbsp oil in a small saucepan. Add the mustard seeds, asafoetida, curry leaves, green chillies and sesame seeds. Let them splutter for 15 seconds.
- Pour this immediately over the besan rolls. Serve hot or at room temperature.

Makkai Squares

(Corn Squares)

Makes 12

Ingredients

2 tsp ghee

100g/3½oz corn kernels, ground

Salt to taste

125g/4½oz boiled peas

3 tbsp refined vegetable oil

8 green chillies, finely chopped

½ tsp cumin seeds

½ tsp mustard seeds

½ tsp garlic paste

½ tbsp ground coriander

½ tbsp ground cumin

175g/6oz maize flour

175g/6oz wholemeal flour

150ml/5fl oz water

Method

- Heat the ghee in a saucepan. When it begins to smoke, fry the corn for 3 minutes. Set aside.
- Add salt to the boiled peas. Mash the peas well. Set aside.
- Heat 2 tbsp oil in a frying pan. Add the green chillies, cumin and mustard seeds. Let them splutter for 15 seconds.
- Add the fried corn, mashed peas, garlic paste, ground coriander and ground cumin. Mix well. Remove from the heat and set aside.
- Mix both the flours together. Add salt and 1 tbsp oil. Add the water and knead into a soft dough.
- Roll out 24 square shapes, each square 10x10cm/4x4in in size.
- Place the corn and peas mixture in the centre of a square and cover with another square. Gently press the edges of the square to seal.
- Repeat for the rest of the squares.
- Grease and heat a frying pan. Roast the squares on the pan till golden brown.
- Serve hot with ketchup.

Dhal Pakwan

(Crispy Bread with Lentils)

Serves 4

Ingredients

600g/1lb 5oz chana dhal*

3 tbsp refined vegetable oil

1 tsp cumin seeds

750ml/1¼ pints water

Salt to taste

½ tsp turmeric

½ tsp amchoor*

10g/¼oz coriander leaves, finely chopped

For the pakwan:

250g/9oz plain white flour

½ tsp cumin seeds

Salt to taste

Refined vegetable oil for deep frying

Method

- Soak the chana dhal for 4 hours. Drain and set aside.
- Heat the oil in a saucepan. Add the cumin seeds. Let them splutter for 15 seconds.
- Add the soaked dhal, water, salt and turmeric. Simmer for 30 minutes.
- Transfer to a serving dish. Sprinkle with the amchoor and coriander leaves. Set aside.
- Knead all the pakwan ingredients, except the oil, with enough water to make a stiff dough.
- Divide into walnut-sized balls. Roll out into thick discs, 10cm/4in in diameter. Pierce all over with a fork.
- Heat the oil in a frying pan. Deep fry the discs till golden. Drain on absorbent paper.
- Serve the pakwans with the hot dhal.

Spicy Sev

(Spicy Gram Flour Flakes)

Serves 4

Ingredients

500g/1lb 2oz besan*

1 tsp ajowan seeds

1 tbsp refined vegetable oil plus extra for deep frying

¼ tsp asafoetida

Salt to taste

200ml/7fl oz water

Method

- Knead the besan with the ajowan seeds, oil, asafoetida, salt and water into a sticky dough.
- Put the dough in a piping bag.
- Heat the oil in a saucepan. Press the dough through the nozzle in the form of noodles into the pan and fry lightly on both sides.
- Drain well and cool before storing.

NOTE: *This can be stored for a fortnight.*

Stuffed Veggie Crescents

Makes 6

Ingredients

350g/12oz plain white flour

6 tbsp warm refined vegetable oil plus extra for deep frying

Salt to taste

1 tomato, sliced

For the filling:

3 tbsp refined vegetable oil

200g/7oz peas

1 carrot, julienned

100g/3½oz French beans, chopped into thin strips

4 tbsp fresh coconut, grated

3 green chillies

2.5cm/1in root ginger, crushed

4 tsp coriander leaves, finely chopped

2 tsp sugar

2 tsp lemon juice

Salt to taste

Method

- First make the filling. Heat the oil in a saucepan. Add the peas, carrot and French beans and fry, stirring continuously, till soft.
- Add all the remaining filling ingredients and mix well. Set aside.
- Mix the flour with the oil and the salt. Knead into a stiff dough.
- Divide the dough into 6 lemon-sized balls.
- Roll each ball into a disc of 10cm/4in diameter.
- Place the vegetable filling on one half of a disc. Fold the other half over to cover the filling and press the edges together to seal.
- Repeat for all the discs.
- Heat the oil in a saucepan. Add the crescents and fry till they are golden brown.
- Arrange them in a round serving dish and garnish with the tomato slices. Serve immediately.

Kachori Usal

(Fried Bread with Chickpeas)

Serves 4

Ingredients
For the pastry:

50g/1¾oz fenugreek leaves finely chopped

175g/6oz wholemeal flour

2 green chillies, finely chopped

1 tsp ginger paste

¼ tsp turmeric

100ml/3½fl oz water

Salt to taste

For the filling:

1 tsp refined vegetable oil

250g/9oz mung beans, boiled

250g/9oz green chickpeas, boiled

¼ tsp turmeric

½ tsp chilli powder

1 tsp ground coriander

1 tsp ground cumin

Salt to taste

For the sauce:

2 tsp refined vegetable oil

2 large onions, finely chopped

2 tomatoes, chopped

1 tsp garlic paste

½ tsp garam masala

¼ tsp chilli powder

Salt to taste

Method

- Mix all the pastry ingredients together. Knead into a firm dough. Set aside.
- For the filling, heat the oil in a frying pan and sauté all the filling ingredients on a medium heat for 5 minutes. Set aside.
- For the sauce, heat the oil in a frying pan. Add all the sauce ingredients. Fry for 5 minutes, stirring occasionally. Set aside.
- Divide the dough into 8 portions. Roll out each portion into a disc of 10cm/4in diameter.
- Place some filling in the centre of a disc. Seal like a pouch and smooth to form a stuffed ball. Repeat for all the discs.

- Steam the balls for 15 minutes.
- Add the balls to the sauce and toss to coat. Cook on a low heat for 5 minutes.
- Serve hot.

Dhal Dhokli

(Gujarati Savoury Snack)

Serves 4

Ingredients
For the dhokli:

175g/6oz wholemeal flour

Pinch of turmeric

¼ tsp chilli powder

½ tsp ajowan seeds

1 tsp refined vegetable oil

100ml/3½fl oz water

For the dhal:

2 tbsp refined vegetable oil

3-4 cloves

5cm/2in cinnamon

1 tsp mustard seeds

300g/10oz masoor dhal*, cooked and mashed

½ tsp turmeric

Pinch of asafoetida

1 tbsp tamarind paste

2 tbsp grated jaggery*

60g/2oz peanuts

1 tsp ground coriander

1 tsp ground cumin

½ tsp chilli powder

Salt to taste

25g/scant 1oz coriander leaves, finely chopped

Method

- Mix all the dhokli ingredients together. Knead to form a firm dough.
- Divide the dough into 5-6 balls. Roll out into thick discs, 6cm/2.4in in diameter. Set aside for 10 minutes to harden.
- Cut out the dhokli discs into diamond-shaped pieces. Set aside.
- For the dhal, heat the oil in a saucepan. Add the cloves, cinnamon and mustard seeds. Let them splutter for 15 seconds.
- Add all the remaining dhal ingredients, except the coriander leaves. Mix well. Cook on a high heat till the dhal starts boiling.
- Add the dhokli pieces to the boiling dhal. Continue to cook over a low heat for 10 minutes.
- Garnish with the coriander leaves. Serve hot.

Misal

(Healthy Sprouted Beans Snack)

Serves 4

Ingredients

3-4 tbsp refined vegetable oil

½ tsp mustard seeds

¼ tsp asafoetida

6 curry leaves

1 tsp ginger paste

1 tsp garlic paste

25g/scant 1oz coriander leaves, ground in a blender

1 tsp chilli powder

1 tsp tamarind paste

2 tsp grated jaggery*

Salt to taste

300g/10oz sprouted mung beans, boiled

2 large potatoes, diced and boiled

500ml/16fl oz water

300g/10oz Bombay Mix*

1 large tomato, finely chopped

1 large onion, finely chopped

25g/scant 1oz coriander leaves, finely chopped

4 slices of bread

For the spice mixture:
1 tsp cumin seeds

2 tsp coriander seeds

2 cloves

3 peppercorns

¼ tsp ground cinnamon

Method

- Grind together all the ingredients of the spice mixture. Set aside.
- Heat the oil in a saucepan. Add the mustard seeds, asafoetida and curry leaves. Let them splutter for 2-3 minutes.
- Add the ginger paste, garlic paste, ground coriander leaves, chilli powder, tamarind paste, jaggery and salt. Mix well and cook for 3-4 minutes.
- Add the ground spice mixture. Sauté for 2-3 minutes.
- Add the sprouted beans, potatoes and water. Mix well and simmer for 15 minutes.
- Transfer to a serving bowl and sprinkle with the Bombay Mix, chopped tomato, chopped onion and coriander leaves on top.
- Serve hot with a slice of bread on the side.

Pandori

(Mung Dhal Snack)

Makes 12

Ingredients

1 green chilli, halved lengthways

Salt to taste

1 tsp bicarbonate of soda

¼ tsp asafoetida

250g/9oz whole mung dhal*, soaked for 4 hours

2 tsp refined vegetable oil

2 tsp coriander leaves, finely chopped

Method

- Add the green chilli, salt, bicarbonate of soda and asafoetida to the dhal. Grind to a paste.
- Grease a 20cm/8in round cake tin with the oil and pour the dhal paste in it. Steam for 10 minutes.
- Set the steamed dhal mixture aside for 10 minutes. Once cool, cut into 2.5cm/1in pieces.
- Garnish with the coriander leaves. Serve hot with green coconut chutney

Vegetable Adai

(Vegetable, Rice and Lentil Crêpe)

Makes 8

Ingredients

100g/3½oz parboiled rice

150g/5½oz masoor dhal*

75g/2½oz urad dhal*

3-4 red chillies

¼ tsp asafoetida

Salt to taste

4 tbsp water

1 onion, finely chopped

½ carrot, finely chopped

50g/1¾oz cabbage,

finely chopped 4-5 curry leaves

10g/¼oz coriander leaves, finely chopped

4 tsp refined vegetable oil

Method

- Soak the rice and the dhals together for about 20 minutes.
- Drain and add the red chillies, asafoetida, salt and water. Grind to a coarse paste.
- Add the onion, carrot, cabbage, curry leaves and coriander leaves. Mix well to make a batter with a consistency similar to sponge cake batter. Add more water if the consistency is not right.
- Grease a flat pan. Pour a spoonful of the batter. Spread with the back of a spoon to make a thin crêpe.
- Pour half a tsp oil around the crêpe. Flip to cook both sides.
- Repeat for the rest of the batter. Serve hot with coconut chutney

Spicy Corn on the Cob

Serves 4

Ingredients

8 corn cobs

Salted butter to taste

Salt to taste

2 tsp chaat masala*

2 lemons, halved

Method

- Roast the corns cobs on a charcoal grill or open flame till golden brown all over.
- Rub the butter, salt, chaat masala and the lemons on each cob.
- Serve immediately.

Mixed Vegetable Chop

Makes 12

Ingredients

Salt to taste

¼ tsp ground black pepper

4-5 large potatoes, boiled and mashed

2 tbsp refined vegetable oil plus extra for deep frying

1 small onion, finely chopped

½ tsp garam masala

1 tsp lemon juice

100g/3½oz frozen mixed vegetables

2-3 green chillies, finely chopped

50g/1¾oz coriander leaves, finely chopped

250g/9oz arrowroot powder

150ml/5fl oz water

100g/3½oz breadcrumbs

Method

- Add the salt and black pepper to the potatoes. Mix well and divide into 12 balls. Set aside.
- For the filling, heat 2 tbsp oil in a frying pan. Fry the onion on a medium heat till translucent.
- Add the garam masala, lemon juice, mixed vegetables, green chillies and coriander leaves. Mix well and cook on a medium heat for 2-3 minutes. Mash well and set aside.
- Flatten the potato balls with greased palms.
- Place some filling mixture on eacn potato patty. Seal to make oblong-shaped chops. Set aside.
- Mix the arrowroot powder with enough water to form a thin batter.
- Heat the oil in a frying pan. Dip the chops in the batter, roll in the breadcrumbs and deep fry on a medium heat till golden brown.
- Drain and serve hot.

Idli Upma

(Steamed Rice Cake Snack)

Serves 4

Ingredients

5 tbsp refined vegetable oil

½ tsp mustard seeds

½ tsp cumin seeds

1 tsp urad dhal*

2 green chillies, slit lengthways

8 curry leaves

Pinch of asafoetida

¼ tsp turmeric

8 idlis crushed

2 tsp caster sugar

1 tbsp coriander leaves, finely chopped

Salt to taste

Method

- Heat the oil in a saucepan. Add the mustard seeds, cumin seeds, urad dhal, green chillies, curry leaves, asafoetida and turmeric. Let them splutter for 30 seconds.
- Add the crushed idlis, caster sugar, coriander and salt. Mix gently.
- Serve immediately.

Dhal Bhajiya

(Batter Fried Lentil Balls)

Makes 15

Ingredients

250/9oz mung dhal*, soaked for 2-3 hours

2 green chillies, finely chopped

2 tbsp coriander leaves, finely chopped

1 tsp cumin seeds

Salt to taste

Refined vegetable oil for deep frying

Method

- Drain the dhal and grind coarsely.
- Add the chillies, coriander leaves, cumin seeds and salt. Mix well.
- Heat the oil in a frying pan. Add small portions of the dhal mixture and fry over a medium heat till golden brown.
- Serve hot with mint chutney

Masala Papad

(Poppadoms Topped with Spices)

Makes 8

Ingredients

2 tomatoes, finely chopped

2 large onions, finely chopped

3 green chillies, finely chopped

10g/¼oz coriander leaves, chopped

2 tsp lemon juice

1 tsp chaat masala*

Salt to taste

8 poppadoms

Method

- Mix all the ingredients, except the poppadoms, in a bowl.
- Roast the poppadoms on a high heat, turning each side. Make sure you don't burn them.
- Spread the vegetable mixture over each poppadom. Serve immediately.

Vegetable Sandwich

Makes 6

Ingredients

12 bread slices

50g/1¾oz butter

100g/3½oz mint chutney

1 large potato, boiled and thinly sliced

1 tomato, thinly sliced

1 large onion, thinly sliced

1 cucumber, thinly sliced

Chaat masala* to taste

Salt to taste

Method

- Butter the bread slices and apply a thin coat of mint chutney on each.
- Place a layer of potato, tomato, onion and cucumber slices on 6 bread slices.
- Sprinkle with some chaat masala and salt.
- Cover with the remaining bread slices and cut as desired. Serve immediately.

Sprouted Mung Bean Rolls

Makes 8

Ingredients

175g/6oz wholemeal flour

2 tbsp plain white flour

½ tsp caster sugar

75ml/ 2½fl oz water

50g/1¾oz frozen peas

25g/scant 1oz sprouted mung beans

2 tbsp refined vegetable oil

50g/1¾oz spinach, finely chopped

1 small tomato, finely chopped

1 small onion, finely chopped

30g/1oz cabbage leaves, finely chopped

1 tsp ground cumin

1 tsp ground coriander

¼ tsp ginger paste

¼ tsp garlic paste

60ml/2fl oz cream

Salt to taste

750g/1lb 10oz yoghurt

Method

- Mix the wholemeal flour, plain white flour, sugar and water. Knead into a stiff dough. Set aside.
- Boil the peas and mung beans in minimum water. Drain and set aside.
- Heat the oil in a saucepan. Add the spinach, tomato, onion and cabbage. Fry, stirring occasionally, till the tomato turns pulpy.
- Add the peas and mung beans mixture along with all remaining ingredients, except the dough. Cook on a medium heat till dry. Set aside.
- Make thin chapattis with the dough.
- On one side of each chapatti, place the cooked mixture lengthways in the centre, and roll up. Serve with mint chutney and yoghurt.

Chutney Sandwich

Makes 6

Ingredients

12 bread slices

½ tsp butter

6 tbsp mint chutney

4 tomatoes, sliced

Method

- Butter all the bread slices. Spread the mint chutney on 6 slices.
- Place the tomatoes over the mint chutney and cover with another buttered slice. Serve immediately.

Chatpata Gobhi

(Tangy Cauliflower Snack)

Serves 4

Ingredients

500g/1lb 2oz cauliflower florets

Salt to taste

1 tsp ground black pepper

1 tbsp refined vegetable oil

1 tbsp lemon juice

Method

- Steam the cauliflower florets for 10 minutes. Set aside to cool.
- Mix the steamed florets thoroughly with the remaining ingredients. Spread the cauliflower on a flameproof dish and grill for 5-7 minutes, or till it turns brown. Serve hot.

Sabudana Vada

(Sago Cutlet)

Makes 12

Ingredients

300g/10oz sago

125g/4½oz peanuts, roasted and crushed coarsely

2 large potatoes, boiled and mashed

5 green chillies, crushed

Salt to taste

Refined vegetable oil for deep frying

Method

- Soak the sago for 5 hours. Drain thoroughly and set aside for 3-4 hours.
- Mix the sago with all the ingredients, except the oil. Knead well.
- Grease your palms and make twelve patties with the mixture.
- Heat the oil in a frying pan. Deep fry 3-4 patties at a time on a medium heat till golden brown.
- Drain on absorbent paper. Serve hot with mint chutney.

Bread Upma

(Bread Snack)

Serves 4

Ingredients

2 tbsp refined vegetable oil

½ tsp mustard seeds

½ tsp cumin seeds

3 green chillies, slit lengthways

½ tsp turmeric

¼ tsp asafoetida

2 onions, finely chopped

2 tomatoes, finely chopped

Salt to taste

2 tsp sugar

3-4 tbsp water

15 bread slices, broken into bits

1 tbsp coriander leaves, chopped

Method

- Heat the oil in a frying pan. Add the mustard seeds, cumin seeds, green chillies, turmeric and asafoetida. Let them splutter for 15 seconds.
- Add the onions and sauté till translucent. Add the tomatoes, salt, sugar and water. Bring to boil on a medium heat.
- Add the bread and mix well. Simmer for 2-3 minutes, stirring occasionally.
- Garnish with the coriander leaves. Serve hot.

Spicy Khaja

(Spicy Flour Dumplings with Ginger)

Makes 25-30

Ingredients

500g/1lb 2oz besan*

85g/3oz plain white flour

2 tsp chilli powder

½ tsp ajowan seeds

½ tsp cumin seeds

1 tbsp coriander leaves, chopped

Salt to taste

200ml/7fl oz water

1 tbsp refined vegetable oil plus extra for deep frying

Method

- Knead all the ingredients, except the oil for frying, into a soft dough.

- Make 25-30 balls of 10cm/4in diameter. Prick all over with a fork.

- Allow to dry on a clean cloth for 25-30 minutes.

- Deep fry till golden brown. Drain, cool and store for up to 15 days.

Crispy Potato

Serves 4

Ingredients

500g/1lb 2oz Greek yoghurt

1 tsp ginger paste

1 tsp garlic paste

1 tsp garam masala

1 tsp ground cumin, dry roasted

1 tbsp mint leaves, chopped

½ tbsp coriander leaves, chopped

Salt to taste

2 tbsp refined vegetable oil

4-5 potatoes, peeled and julienned

Method

- Whisk the yoghurt in a bowl. Add all the ingredients, except the oil and the potatoes. Mix well.

- Marinate the potatoes with the yoghurt for 3-4 hours in the refrigerator.

- Pour the oil in a grilling pan and arrange the marinated potatoes on it.

- Grill for 10 minutes. Turn the potatoes and grill for another 8-10 minutes till crispy. Serve hot.

Dhal Vada

(Fried Mixed Lentil Patties)

Makes 15

Ingredients

300g/10oz whole masoor dhal*

150g/5½oz masoor dhal*

1 large onion, finely chopped

2.5cm/1in root ginger, finely chopped

3 green chillies, finely chopped

¼ tbsp asafoetida

Salt to taste

Refined vegetable oil for frying

Method

- Mix the dhals together. Place in a colander and pour water in them. Set aside for an hour. Pat dry with a towel.

- Grind the dhals into a paste. Add all the remaining ingredients, except the oil. Mix well and shape the mixture into patties.

- Heat the oil in a frying pan. Deep fry the patties on a medium heat till golden brown. Serve hot with mint chutney

Zunka

(Spicy Gram Flour Curry)

Serves 4

Ingredients

750g/1lb 10oz besan*, dry roasted

400ml/14fl oz water

4 tbsp refined vegetable oil

½ tsp mustard seeds

½ tsp cumin seeds

½ tsp turmeric

3-4 green chillies, slit lengthways

10 garlic cloves, crushed

3 small onions, finely chopped

1 tsp tamarind paste

Salt to taste

Method

- Mix the besan with enough water to form a thick paste. Set aside.

- Heat the oil in a saucepan. Add the mustard and cumin seeds. Let them splutter for 15 seconds. Add the remaining ingredients. Fry for a minute. Add the besan paste and stir continuously on a low heat till thick. Serve hot.

Turnip Curry

Serves 4

Ingredients

3 tsp poppy seeds

3 tsp sesame seeds

3 tsp coriander seeds

3 tsp fresh coconut, grated

125g/4½oz yoghurt

120ml/4fl oz refined vegetable oil

2 large onions, finely chopped

1½ tsp chilli powder

1 tsp ginger paste

1 tsp garlic paste

400g/14oz turnips, chopped

Salt to taste

Method

- Dry roast the poppy, sesame and coriander seeds and the coconut for 1-2 minutes. Grind to a paste.

- Whisk this paste with the yoghurt. Set aside.

- Heat the oil in a saucepan. Add the remaining ingredients. Fry them on a medium heat for 5 minutes. Add the yoghurt mixture. Simmer for 7-8 minutes. Serve hot.

Chhaner Dhalna

(Bengali Style Paneer)

Serves 4

Ingredients

2 tbsp mustard oil plus extra for deep frying

225g/8oz paneer*, diced

2.5cm/1in cinnamon

3 green cardamom pods

4 cloves

½ tsp cumin seeds

1 tsp turmeric

2 large potatoes, diced and fried

½ tsp chilli powder

2 tsp sugar

Salt to taste

250ml/8fl oz water

2 tbsp coriander leaves, chopped

Method

- Heat the oil for deep frying in a frying pan. Add the paneer and fry on a medium heat till golden brown. Drain and set aside.

- Heat the remaining oil in a saucepan. Add the remaining ingredients, except the water and coriander leaves. Fry for 2-3 minutes.

- Add the water. Simmer for 7-8 minutes. Add the paneer. Simmer for 5 more minutes. Garnish with the coriander leaves. Serve hot.

Corn with Coconut

Serves 4

Ingredients

2 tbsp ghee

600g/1lb 5oz corn kernels, cooked

1 tsp sugar

1 tsp salt

10g/¼oz coriander leaves, finely chopped

For the coconut paste:

50g/1¾oz fresh coconut, grated

3 tbsp poppy seeds

1 tsp coriander seeds

2.5cm/1in root ginger, julienned

3 green chillies

125g/4½oz peanuts

Method

- Coarsely grind all the ingredients for the coconut paste. Heat the ghee in a frying pan. Add the paste and fry for 4-5 minutes, stirring continuously.

- Add the corn, sugar and salt. Cook on a low heat for 4-5 minutes.

- Garnish with the coriander leaves. Serve hot.

Green Pepper with Potato

Serves 4

Ingredients

2 tbsp refined vegetable oil

1 tsp cumin seeds

10 garlic cloves, finely chopped

3 large potatoes, diced

2 tsp ground coriander

1 tsp ground cumin

½ tsp turmeric

½ tsp amchoor[*]

½ tsp garam masala

Salt to taste

3 large green peppers, julienned

3 tbsp coriander leaves, chopped

Method

- Heat the oil in a saucepan. Add the cumin seeds and garlic. Fry for 30 seconds.

- Add the remaining ingredients, except the peppers and coriander leaves. Stir-fry on a medium heat for 5-6 minutes.

- Add the peppers. Stir-fry on a low heat for 5 more minutes. Garnish with the coriander leaves. Serve hot.

Spicy Peas with Potatoes

Serves 4

Ingredients

2 tbsp refined vegetable oil

1 tsp ginger paste

1 large onion, finely chopped

2 large potatoes, diced

500g/1lb 2oz canned peas

½ tsp turmeric

Salt to taste

½ tsp garam masala

2 large tomatoes, diced

½ tsp chilli powder

1 tsp sugar

1 tbsp coriander leaves, chopped

Method

- Heat the oil in a saucepan. Add the ginger paste and onion. Fry them till the onion is translucent.

- Add the remaining ingredients, except the coriander leaves. Mix well. Cover with a lid and cook on a low heat for 10 minutes.

- Garnish with the coriander leaves. Serve hot.

Sautéed Mushrooms

Serves 4

Ingredients

2 tbsp refined vegetable oil

4 green chillies, slit lengthways

8 garlic cloves, crushed

100g/3½oz green peppers, sliced

400g/14oz mushrooms, sliced

Salt to taste

½ tsp coarsely ground black pepper

25g/scant 1oz coriander leaves, chopped

Method

- Heat the oil in a frying pan. Add the green chillies, garlic and green peppers. Fry them on a medium heat for 1-2 minutes.

- Add the mushrooms, salt and pepper. Mix well. Sauté on a medium heat till tender. Garnish with the coriander leaves. Serve hot.

Spicy Mushroom with Baby Corn

Serves 4

Ingredients

2 tbsp refined vegetable oil

1 tsp cumin seeds

2 bay leaves

1 tsp ginger paste

2 green chillies, finely chopped

1 large onion, finely chopped

200g/7oz mushrooms, halved

8-10 baby corns, chopped

125g/4½oz tomato purée

½ tsp turmeric

Salt to taste

½ tsp garam masala

½ tsp sugar

10g/¼oz coriander leaves, chopped

Method

- Heat the oil in a saucepan. Add the cumin seeds and bay leaves. Let them splutter for 15 seconds.

- Add the ginger paste, green chillies and onion. Sauté for 1-2 minutes.

- Add the remaining ingredients, except the coriander leaves. Mix well. Cover with a lid and cook on a low heat for 10 minutes.

- Garnish with the coriander leaves. Serve hot.

Dry Spicy Cauliflower

Serves 4

Ingredients

750g/1lb 10oz cauliflower florets

Salt to taste

Pinch of turmeric

4 bay leaves

750ml/1¼ pints water

2 tbsp refined vegetable oil

4 cloves

4 green cardamom pods

1 large onion, sliced

1 tsp ginger paste

1 tsp garlic paste

1 tsp garam masala

½ tsp chilli powder

¼ tsp ground black pepper

10 cashew nuts, ground

2 tbsp yoghurt

3 tbsp tomato purée

3 tbsp butter

60ml/2fl oz single cream

Method

- Cook the cauliflower with the salt, turmeric, bay leaves and water in a saucepan on a medium heat for 10 minutes. Drain and arrange the florets in an ovenproof dish. Set aside.

- Heat the oil in a saucepan. Add the cloves and cardamom. Let them splutter for 15 seconds.

- Add the onion, ginger paste and garlic paste. Fry for a minute.

- Add the garam masala, chilli powder, pepper and cashew nuts. Fry for 1-2 minutes.

- Add the yoghurt and tomato purée. Mix thoroughly. Add the butter and cream. Stir for a minute. Remove from the heat.

- Pour this over the cauliflower florets. Bake at 150°C (300°F, Gas Mark 2) in a pre-heated oven for 8-10 minutes. Serve hot.

Mushroom Curry

Serves 4

Ingredients

3 tbsp refined vegetable oil

2 large onions, grated

1 tsp ginger paste

1 tsp garlic paste

½ tsp turmeric

1 tsp chilli powder

1 tsp ground coriander

400g/14oz mushrooms, quartered

200g/7oz peas

2 tomatoes, finely chopped

½ tsp garam masala

Salt to taste

20 cashew nuts, ground

240ml/6fl oz water

Method

- Heat the oil in a saucepan. Add the onions. Fry them till they are brown.

- Add the ginger paste, garlic paste, turmeric, chilli powder and ground coriander. Sauté on a medium heat for a minute.

- Add the remaining ingredients. Mix well. Cover with a lid and simmer for 8-10 minutes. Serve hot.

Baingan Bharta

(Roasted Aubergine)

Serves 4

Ingredients

- 1 large aubergine
- 3 tbsp refined vegetable oil
- 1 large onion, finely chopped
- 3 green chillies, slit lengthways
- ¼ tsp turmeric
- Salt to taste
- ½ tsp garam masala
- 1 tomato, finely chopped

Method

- Pierce the aubergine all over with a fork and grill it for 25 minutes. Once it has cooled, discard the roasted skin and mash the flesh. Set aside.

- Heat the oil in a saucepan. Add the onion and green chillies. Fry on a medium heat for 2 minutes.

- Add the turmeric, salt, garam masala and tomato. Mix well. Fry for 5 minutes. Add the mashed aubergine. Mix well.

- Cook on a low heat for 8 minutes, stirring occasionally. Serve hot.

Vegetable Hyderabadi

Serves 4

Ingredients

2 tbsp refined vegetable oil

½ tsp mustard seeds

1 large onion, finely chopped

400g/14oz frozen, mixed vegetables

½ tsp turmeric

Salt to taste

For the spice mixture:

2.5cm/1in root ginger

8 garlic cloves

2 cloves

2.5cm/1in cinnamon

1 tsp fenugreek seeds

3 green chillies

4 tbsp fresh coconut, grated

10 cashew nuts

Method

- Grind all the ingredients of the spice mixture together. Set aside.

- Heat the oil in a saucepan. Add the mustard seeds. Let them splutter for 15 seconds. Add the onion and fry till brown.

- Add the remaining ingredients and the ground spice mixture. Mix well. Cook on a low heat for 8-10 minutes. Serve hot.

Kaddu Bhaji*

(Dry Red Pumpkin)

Serves 4

Ingredients

3 tbsp refined vegetable oil

½ tsp cumin seeds

¼ tsp fenugreek seeds

600g/1lb 5oz pumpkin, thinly sliced

Salt to taste

½ tsp roasted ground cumin

½ tsp chilli powder

¼ tsp turmeric

1 tsp amchoor*

1 tsp sugar

Method

- Heat the oil in a saucepan. Add the cumin and fenugreek seeds. Let them splutter for 15 seconds. Add the pumpkin and salt. Mix well. Cover with a lid and cook on a medium heat for 8 minutes.

- Uncover and lightly crush with the back of a spoon. Add the remaining ingredients. Mix well. Cook for 5 minutes. Serve hot.

Muthia nu Shak

(Fenugreek Dumplings in Sauce)

Serves 4

Ingredients

200g/7oz fresh fenugreek leaves, finely chopped

Salt to taste

125g/4½oz wholemeal flour

125g/4½oz besan*

2 green chillies, finely chopped

1 tsp ginger paste

3 tsp sugar

Juice of 1 lemon

½ tsp garam masala

½ tsp turmeric

Pinch of bicarbonate of soda

3 tbsp refined vegetable oil

½ tsp ajowan seeds

½ tsp mustard seeds

Pinch of asafoetida

250ml/8fl oz water

Method

- Mix the fenugreek leaves with the salt. Set aside for 10 minutes. Squeeze out the moisture.

- Mix the fenugreek leaves with the flour, besan, green chillies, ginger paste, sugar, lemon juice, garam masala, turmeric and bicarbonate of soda. Knead into a soft dough.

- Divide the dough into 30 walnut-sized balls. Flatten slightly to form the muthias. Set aside.

- Heat the oil in a saucepan. Add the ajowan seeds, mustard seeds and asafoetida. Let them splutter for 15 seconds.

- Add the muthias and water.

- Cover with a lid and simmer for 10-15 minutes. Serve hot.

Pumpkin Koot

(Pumpkin in Lentil Curry)

Serves 4

Ingredients

50g/1¾oz fresh coconut, grated

1 tsp cumin seeds

2 red chillies

150g/5½oz mung dhal*, soaked for 30 minutes and drained

2 tbsp chana dhal*

Salt to taste

500ml/16fl oz water

2 tbsp refined vegetable oil

250g/9oz pumpkin, diced

¼ tsp turmeric

Method

- Grind the coconut, cumin seeds and red chillies to a paste. Set aside.

- Mix the dhals with the salt and water. Cook this mixture in a saucepan on a medium heat for 40 minutes. Set aside.

- Heat the oil in a saucepan. Add the pumpkin, turmeric, boiled dhals and the coconut paste. Mix well. Simmer for 10 minutes. Serve hot.

Rassa

(Cauliflower and Peas in Sauce)

Serves 4

Ingredients

2 tbsp refined vegetable oil plus extra for deep frying

250g/9oz cauliflower florets

2 tbsp fresh coconut, grated

1cm/½in root ginger, crushed

4-5 green chillies, slit lengthways

2-3 tomatoes, finely chopped

400g/14oz frozen peas

1 tsp sugar

Salt to taste

Method

- Heat the oil for deep frying in a saucepan. Add the cauliflower. Deep fry on a medium heat till golden brown. Drain and set aside.
- Grind the coconut, ginger, green chillies and tomatoes. Heat 2 tbsp oil in a saucepan. Add this paste and fry for 1-2 minutes.
- Add the cauliflower and the remaining ingredients. Mix well. Cook on a low heat for 4-5 minutes. Serve hot.

Doodhi Manpasand

(Bottle Gourd in Sauce)

Serves 4

Ingredients

3 tbsp refined vegetable oil

3 dried red chillies

1 large onion, finely chopped

500g/1lb 2oz bottle gourd*, chopped

¼ tsp turmeric

2 tsp ground coriander

1 tsp ground cumin

½ tsp chilli powder

½ tsp garam masala

2.5cm/1in root ginger, finely chopped

2 tomatoes, finely chopped

1 green pepper, cored, deseeded and finely chopped

Salt to taste

2 tsp coriander leaves, finely chopped

Method

- Heat the oil in a saucepan. Fry the red chillies and onion for 2 minutes.
- Add the remaining ingredients, except the coriander leaves. Mix well. Cook on a low heat for 5-7 minutes. Garnish with the coriander leaves. Serve hot.

Tomato Chokha

(Tomato Compote)

Serves 4

Ingredients

6 large tomatoes

2 tbsp refined vegetable oil

1 big onion, finely chopped

8 garlic cloves, finely chopped

1 green chilli, finely chopped

½ tsp chilli powder

10g/¼oz coriander leaves, finely chopped

Salt to taste

Method

- Grill the tomatoes for 10 minutes. Peel and crush to a pulp. Set aside.
- Heat the oil in a saucepan. Add the onion, garlic and green chilli. Fry for 2-3 minutes. Add the remaining ingredients and the tomato pulp. Mix well. Cover with a lid and cook for 5-6 minutes. Serve hot.

Baingan Chokha

(Aubergine Compote)

Serves 4

Ingredients

1 large aubergine

2 tbsp refined vegetable oil

1 small onion, chopped

8 garlic cloves, finely chopped

1 green chilli, finely chopped

1 tomato, finely chopped

60g/2oz corn kernels, boiled

10g/¼oz coriander leaves, finely chopped

Salt to taste

Method

- Pierce the aubergine all over with a fork. Grill for 10-15 minutes. Peel and crush to a pulp. Set aside.
- Heat the oil in a saucepan. Add the onion, garlic and green chilli. Fry them on a medium heat for 5 minutes.
- Add the remaining ingredients and the aubergine pulp. Mix well. Cook for 3-4 minutes. Serve hot.

Cauliflower & Peas Curry

Serves 4

Ingredients

3 tbsp refined vegetable oil

¼ tsp turmeric

3 green chillies, slit lengthways

1 tsp ground coriander

2.5cm/1in root ginger, grated

250g/9oz cauliflower florets

400g/14oz fresh green peas

60ml/2fl oz water

Salt to taste

1 tbsp coriander leaves, finely chopped

Method

- Heat the oil in a saucepan. Add the turmeric, green chillies, ground coriander and ginger. Fry on a medium heat for a minute.
- Add the remaining ingredients, except the coriander leaves. Mix well Simmer for 10 minutes.
- Garnish with the coriander leaves. Serve hot.

Aloo Methi ki Sabzi

(Potato and Fenugreek Curry)

Serves 4

Ingredients

100g/3½oz fenugreek leaves, chopped

Salt to taste

4 tbsp refined vegetable oil

1 tsp cumin seeds

5-6 green chillies

¼ tsp turmeric

Pinch of asafoetida

6 large potatoes, boiled and chopped

Method

- Mix the fenugreek leaves with the salt. Set aside for 10 minutes.
- Heat the oil in a saucepan. Add the cumin seeds, chillies and turmeric. Let them splutter for 15 seconds.
- Add the remaining ingredients and the fenugreek leaves. Mix well. Cook for 8-10 minutes on a low heat. Serve hot.

Sweet & Sour Karela

Serves 4

Ingredients

500g/1lb 2oz bitter gourds*

Salt to taste

750ml/1¼ pints water

1cm/½in root ginger

10 garlic cloves

4 large onions, chopped

4 tbsp refined vegetable oil

Pinch of asafoetida

½ tsp turmeric

1 tsp ground coriander

1 tsp ground cumin

1 tsp tamarind paste

2 tbsp jaggery*, grated

Method

- Peel the bitter gourds. Slice and soak them in salty water for 1 hour. Rinse and squeeze out the excess water. Wash and set aside.
- Grind the ginger, garlic and onions to a paste. Set aside.
- Heat the oil in a saucepan. Add the asafoetida. Let it splutter for 15 seconds. Add the ginger-onion paste and the remaining ingredients. Mix well. Fry for 3-4 minutes. Add the bitter gourds. Mix well. Cover with a lid and cook on a low heat for 8-10 minutes. Serve hot.

Karela Koshimbir

(Crispy Crushed Bitter Gourd)

Serves 4

Ingredients

500g/1lb 2oz bitter gourds*, peeled

Salt to taste

Refined vegetable oil for frying

2 medium-sized onions, chopped

50g/1¾oz coriander leaves, chopped

3 green chillies, finely chopped

½ fresh coconut, grated

1 tbsp lemon juice

Method

- Slice the bitter gourds. Rub the salt on them and set aside for 2-3 hours.
- Heat the oil in a saucepan. Add the bitter gourds and fry on a medium heat till brown and crispy. Drain, cool a little and crush with your fingers.
- Mix the remaining ingredients in a bowl. Add the gourds and serve while they are still warm.

Karela Curry

(Bitter Gourd Curry)

Serves 4

Ingredients

½ coconut

2 red chillies

1 tsp cumin seeds

3 tbsp refined vegetable oil

1 pinch of asafoetida

2 large onions, finely chopped

2 green chillies, finely chopped

Salt to taste

½ tsp turmeric

500g/1lb 2oz bitter gourds*, peeled and chopped

2 tomatoes, finely chopped

Method

- Grate half of the coconut and chop the rest. Set aside.
- Dry roast (see cooking techniques) the grated coconut, red chillies and cumin seeds. Cool and grind together to a fine paste. Set aside.
- Heat the oil in a frying pan. Add the asafoetida, onions, green chillies, salt, turmeric and chopped coconut. Fry for 3 minutes, stirring frequently.
- Add the bitter gourds and tomatoes. Cook for 3-4 minutes.
- Add the ground coconut paste. Cook for 5-7 minutes and serve hot.

Chilli Cauliflower

Serves 4

Ingredients

3 tbsp refined vegetable oil

5cm/2in root ginger, finely chopped

12 garlic cloves, finely chopped

1 cauliflower, chopped into florets

5 red chillies, quartered and deseeded

6 spring onions, halved

3 tomatoes, blanched and chopped

Salt to taste

Method

- Heat the oil in a saucepan. Add the ginger and garlic. Fry on a medium heat for a minute.
- Add the cauliflower and red chillies. Stir-fry for 5 minutes.
- Add the remaining ingredients. Mix well. Cook on a low heat for 7-8 minutes. Serve hot.

Nutty Curry

Serves 4

Ingredients

4 tbsp ghee

10g/¼oz cashew nuts

10g/¼oz almonds, blanched

10-12 peanuts

5-6 raisins

10 pistachios

10 walnuts, chopped

2.5cm/1in root ginger, grated

6 garlic cloves, crushed

4 small onions, finely chopped

4 tomatoes, finely chopped

4 dates, de-seeded and sliced

½ tsp turmeric

125g/4½oz khoya*

1 tsp garam masala

Salt to taste

75g/2½ Cheddar cheese, grated

1 tbsp coriander leaves, chopped

Method

- Heat the ghee in a frying pan. Add all the nuts and fry them on a medium heat till they turn golden brown. Drain and set aside.
- In the same ghee, fry the ginger, garlic and onion till brown.
- Add the fried nuts and all the remaining ingredients, except the cheese and coriander leaves. Cover with a lid. Cook on a low heat for 5 minutes.
- Garnish with the cheese and coriander leaves. Serve hot.

Daikon Leaves Bhaaji

Serves 4

Ingredients

2 tbsp refined vegetable oil

¼ tsp ground cumin

2 red chillies, broken into bits

Pinch of asafoetida

400g/14oz daikon leaves*, chopped

300g/10oz chana dhal*, soaked for 1 hour

1 tsp jaggery*, grated

¼ tsp turmeric

Salt to taste

Method

- Heat the oil in a saucepan. Add the cumin, red chillies and asafoetida.
- Let them splutter for 15 seconds. Add the remaining ingredients. Mix well. Cook on a low heat for 10-15 minutes. Serve hot.

Chhole Aloo

(Chickpea and Potato Curry)

Serves 4

Ingredients

500g/1lb 2oz chickpeas, soaked overnight

Pinch of bicarbonate of soda

Salt to taste

1 litre/1¾ pints water

3 tbsp ghee

2.5cm/1in root ginger, julienned

2 large onions, grated, plus 1 small onion, sliced

2 tomatoes, diced

1 tsp garam masala

1 tsp ground cumin, dry roasted (see cooking techniques)

½ tsp ground green cardamom

½ tsp turmeric

2 large potatoes, boiled and diced

2 tsp tamarind paste

1 tbsp coriander leaves, chopped

Method

- Cook the chickpeas with the bicarbonate of soda, salt and water in a saucepan on a medium heat for 45 minutes. Drain and set aside.
- Heat the ghee in a saucepan. Add the ginger and grated onions. Fry till translucent. Add the remaining ingredients, except the coriander leaves and sliced onion. Mix well. Add the chickpeas and cook for 7-8 minutes.
- Garnish with the coriander leaves and sliced onion. Serve hot.

Peanut Curry

Serves 4

Ingredients

1 tsp poppy seeds

1 tsp coriander seeds

1 tsp cumin seeds

2 red chillies

25g/scant 1oz fresh coconut, grated

3 tbsp ghee

2 small onions, grated

900g/2lb peanuts, pounded

1 tsp amchoor*

½ tsp turmeric

1 big tomato, blanched and chopped

2 tsp jaggery*, grated

500ml/16fl oz water

Salt to taste

15g/½oz coriander leaves, chopped

Method

- Grind the poppy seeds, coriander seeds, cumin seeds, red chillies and coconut to a fine paste. Set aside.
- Heat the ghee in a saucepan. Add the onions. Fry till translucent.
- Add the ground paste and the remaining ingredients, except the coriander leaves. Mix well. Simmer for 7-8 minutes.
- Garnish with the coriander leaves. Serve hot.

French Beans Upkari

(French Beans with Coconut)

Serves 4

Ingredients

1 tbsp refined vegetable oil

½ tsp mustard seeds

½ tsp urad dhal*

2-3 red chillies, broken

500g/1lb 2oz French beans, chopped

1 tsp jaggery*, grated

Salt to taste

25g/scant 1oz fresh coconut, grated

Method

- Heat the oil in a saucepan. Add the mustard seeds. Let them splutter for 15 seconds.
- Add the dhal. Fry till golden brown. Add the remaining ingredients, except the coconut. Mix well. Cook on a low heat for 8-10 minutes.
- Garnish with the coconut. Serve hot.

Karatey Ambadey

(Bitter Gourd and Unripe Mango Curry)

Serves 4

Ingredients

250g/9oz bitter gourd*, sliced

Salt to taste

60g/2oz jaggery*, grated

1 tsp refined vegetable oil

4 dry red chillies

1 tsp urad dhal*

1 tsp fenugreek seeds

2 tsp coriander seeds

50g/1¾oz fresh coconut, grated

¼ tsp turmeric

4 small unripe mangoes

Method

- Rub the bitter gourd pieces with the salt. Set aside for an hour.
- Squeeze out the water from the gourd pieces. Cook them in a saucepan with the jaggery on a medium heat for 4-5 minutes. Set aside.
- Heat the oil in a saucepan. Add the red chillies, dhal, fenugreek and coriander seeds. Fry for a minute. Add the bitter gourd and the remaining ingredients. Mix well. Cook on a low heat for 4-5 minutes. Serve hot.

Kadhai Paneer

(Spicy Paneer)

Serves 4

Ingredients

2 tbsp refined vegetable oil

1 large onion, sliced

3 large green peppers, finely chopped

500g/1lb 2oz paneer*, chopped into 2.5cm/1in pieces

1 tomato, finely chopped

¼ tsp ground coriander, dry roasted (see cooking techniques)

Salt to taste

10g/¼oz coriander leaves, chopped

Method

- Heat the oil in a saucepan. Add the onion and peppers. Fry on a medium heat for 2-3 minutes.
- Add the remaining ingredients, except the coriander leaves. Mix well. Cook on a low heat for 5 minutes. Garnish with the coriander leaves. Serve hot.

Kathirikkai Vangi

(South Indian Aubergine Curry)

Serves 4

Ingredients

150g/5½oz masoor dhal*

Salt to taste

¼ tsp turmeric

500ml/16fl oz water

250g/9oz thin aubergines, sliced

1 tsp refined vegetable oil

¼ tsp mustard seeds

1 tsp tamarind paste

8-10 curry leaves

1 tsp sambhar powder*

Method

- Mix the masoor dhal with salt, a pinch of turmeric and half the water. Cook in a saucepan on a medium heat for 40 minutes. Set aside.
- Cook the aubergines with salt and the remaining turmeric and water in another saucepan on a medium heat for 20 minutes. Set aside.
- Heat the oil in a saucepan. Add the mustard seeds. Let them splutter for 15 seconds. Add the remaining ingredients, the dhal and the aubergine. Mix well. Simmer for 6-7 minutes. Serve hot.

Pitla

(Spicy Gram Flour Curry)

Serves 4

Ingredients

250g/9oz besan*

500ml/16fl oz water

2 tbsp refined vegetable oil

¼ tsp mustard seeds

2 large onions, finely chopped

6 garlic cloves, crushed

2 tbsp tamarind paste

1 tsp garam masala

Salt to taste

1 tbsp coriander leaves, chopped

Method
- Mix the besan and the water. Set aside.
- Heat the oil in a saucepan. Add the mustard seeds. Let them splutter for 15 seconds. Add the onions and garlic. Fry till the onions are brown.
- Add the besan paste. Cook on a low heat till it starts to boil.
- Add the remaining ingredients. Simmer for 5 minutes. Serve hot.

Cauliflower Masala

Serves 4

Ingredients

1 large cauliflower, parboiled (see cooking techniques) in salted water

3 tbsp refined vegetable oil

2 tbsp coriander leaves, finely chopped

1 tsp ground coriander

½ tsp ground cumin

¼ tsp ground ginger

Salt to taste

120ml/4fl oz water

For the sauce:

200g/7oz yoghurt

1 tbsp besan*, dry roasted (see cooking techniques)

¾ tsp chilli powder

Method

- Drain the cauliflower and chop into florets.
- Heat 2 tbsp oil in a frying pan. Add the cauliflower and fry it on a medium heat till golden brown. Set aside.
- Mix all the sauce ingredients together.
- Heat 1 tbsp oil in a saucepan and add this mixture. Fry for a minute.
- Cover with a lid and simmer for 8-10 minutes.
- Add the cauliflower. Mix well. Simmer for 5 minutes.
- Garnish with the coriander leaves. Serve hot.

Shukna Kacha Pepe

(Green Papaya Curry)

Serves 4

Ingredients

150g/5½oz chana dhal*, soaked overnight, drained and ground to a paste

3 tbsp refined vegetable oil plus for deep frying

2 whole dry red chillies

½ tsp fenugreek seeds

½ tsp mustard seeds

1 unripe papaya, peeled and grated

1 tsp turmeric

1 tbsp sugar

Salt to taste

Method

- Divide the dhal paste into walnut-sized balls. Flatten into thin discs.
- Heat the oil for deep frying in a frying pan. Add the discs. Deep fry on a medium heat till golden brown. Drain and break into small pieces. Set aside.
- Heat the remaining oil in a saucepan. Add the chillies, fenugreek and mustard seeds. Let them splutter for 15 seconds.
- Add the remaining ingredients. Mix well. Cover with a lid and cook on a low heat for 8-10 minutes. Add the dhal pieces. Mix well and serve.

Dry Okra

Serves 4

Ingredients

3 tbsp mustard oil

½ tsp kalonji seeds*

750g/1lb 10oz okra, slit lengthways

Salt to taste

½ tsp chilli powder

½ tsp turmeric

2 tsp sugar

3 tsp ground mustard

1 tbsp tamarind paste

Method

- Heat the oil in a saucepan. Fry the onion seeds and okra for 5 minutes.
- Add the salt, chilli powder, turmeric and sugar. Cover with a lid. Cook on a low heat for 10 minutes.
- Add the remaining ingredients. Mix well. Cook for 2-3 minutes. Serve hot.

Moghlai Cauliflower

Serves 4

Ingredients

5cm/2in root ginger

2 tsp cumin seeds

6-7 black peppercorns

500g/1lb 2oz cauliflower florets

Salt to taste

2 tbsp ghee

2 bay leaves

200g/7oz yoghurt

500ml/16fl oz coconut milk

1 tsp sugar

Method

- Grind the ginger, cumin seeds and peppercorns to a fine paste.
- Marinate the cauliflower florets with this paste and salt for 20 minutes.
- Heat the ghee in a frying pan. Add the florets. Fry till golden brown. Add the remaining ingredients. Mix well. Cover with a lid and simmer for 7-8 minutes. Serve hot.

Bhapa Shorshe Baingan

(Aubergine in Mustard Sauce)

Serves 4

Ingredients

- 2 long aubergines
- Salt to taste
- ¼ tsp turmeric
- 3 tbsp refined vegetable oil
- 3 tbsp mustard oil
- 2–3 tbsp ready-made mustard
- 1 tbsp coriander leaves, finely chopped
- 1-2 green chillies, finely chopped

Method

- Slice each aubergine lengthways into 8-12 pieces. Marinate with the salt and turmeric for 5 minutes.
- Heat the oil in a saucepan. Add the aubergine slices and cover with a lid. Cook on a medium heat for 3-4 minutes, turning occasionally.
- Whisk the mustard oil with the ready-made mustard and add to the aubergines. Mix well. Cook on a medium heat for a minute.
- Garnish with the coriander leaves and green chillies. Serve hot.

Baked Vegetables in Spicy Sauce

Serves 4

Ingredients

2 tbsp butter

4 garlic cloves, finely chopped

1 large onion, finely chopped

1 tbsp plain white flour

200g/7oz frozen mixed vegetables

Salt to taste

1 tsp chilli powder

1 tsp mustard paste

250ml/8fl oz ketchup

4 large potatoes, boiled and sliced

250ml/8fl oz white sauce

4 tbsp grated Cheddar cheese

Method

- Heat the butter in a saucepan. Add the garlic and onion. Fry till translucent. Add the flour and fry for a minute.
- Add the vegetables, salt, chilli powder, mustard paste and ketchup. Cook on a medium heat for 4-5 minutes. Set aside.
- Grease a baking dish. Arrange the vegetable mixture and the potatoes in alternate layers. Pour the white sauce and cheese on top.
- Bake in an oven at 200°C (400°F, Gas Mark 6) for 20 minutes. Serve hot.

Tasty Tofu

Serves 4

Ingredients

2 tbsp refined vegetable oil

3 small onions, grated

1 tsp ginger paste

1 tsp garlic paste

3 tomatoes, puréed

50g/1¾oz Greek yoghurt, whisked

400g/14oz tofu, chopped into 2.5cm/1in pieces

25g/scant 1oz coriander leaves, finely chopped

Salt to taste

Method

- Heat the oil in a saucepan. Add the onions, ginger paste and garlic paste. Stir-fry for 5 minutes on a medium heat.
- Add the remaining ingredients. Mix well. Simmer for 3-4 minutes. Serve hot.

Aloo Baingan

(Potato and Aubergine Curry)

Serves 4

Ingredients

3 tbsp refined vegetable oil

1 tsp mustard seeds

½ tsp asafoetida

1cm/½in root ginger, finely chopped

4 green chillies, slit lengthways

10 garlic cloves, finely chopped

6 curry leaves

½ tsp turmeric

3 large potatoes, boiled and diced

250g/9oz aubergines, chopped

½ tsp amchoor*

Salt to taste

Method

- Heat the oil in a saucepan. Add the mustard seeds and asafoetida. Let them splutter for 15 seconds.
- Add the ginger, green chillies, garlic and curry leaves. Fry for 1 minute, stirring continuously.
- Add the remaining ingredients. Mix well. Cover with a lid and simmer for 10-12 minutes. Serve hot.

Sugar Snap Pea Curry

Serves 4

Ingredients

500g/1lb 2oz sugar snap peas

2 tbsp refined vegetable oil

1 tsp ginger paste

1 large onion, finely chopped

2 large potatoes, peeled and diced

½ tsp turmeric

½ tsp garam masala

½ tsp chilli powder

1 tsp sugar

2 large tomatoes, diced

Salt to taste

Method

- Peel the strings from the edges of the pea pods. Chop the pods. Set aside.
- Heat the oil in a saucepan. Add the ginger paste and onion. Fry till translucent. Add the remaining ingredients and the pods. Mix well. Cover with a lid and cook on a low heat for 7-8 minutes. Serve hot.

Potato Pumpkin Curry

Serves 4

Ingredients

2 tbsp refined vegetable oil

1 tsp panch phoron*

Pinch of asafoetida

1 dried red chilli, broken into bits

1 bay leaf

4 large potatoes, diced

200g/7oz pumpkin, diced

½ tsp ginger paste

½ tsp garlic paste

1 tsp ground cumin

1 tsp ground coriander

¼ tsp turmeric

½ tsp garam masala

1 tsp amchoor*

500ml/16fl oz water

Salt to taste

Method

- Heat the oil in a saucepan. Add the panch phoron. Let them splutter for 15 seconds.
- Add the asafoetida, red chilli pieces and the bay leaf. Fry for a minute.
- Add the remaining ingredients. Mix well. Simmer for 10-12 minutes. Serve hot.

Egg Thoran

(Spicy Scrambled Egg)

Serves 4

Ingredients

60ml/2fl oz refined vegetable oil

¼ tsp mustard seeds

2 onions, finely chopped

1 large tomato, finely chopped

1 tsp freshly ground black pepper

Salt to taste

4 eggs, whisked

25g/scant 1oz fresh coconut, grated

50g/1¾oz coriander leaves, chopped

Method

- Heat the oil in a saucepan and fry the mustard seeds. Let them splutter for 15 seconds. Add the onions and fry till brown. Add the tomato, pepper and salt. Fry for 2-3 minutes.
- Add the eggs. Cook on a low heat, scrambling continuously.
- Garnish with the coconut and coriander leaves. Serve hot.

Baingan Lajawab

(Aubergine with Cauliflower)

Serves 4

Ingredients

4 large aubergines

2 tbsp refined vegetable oil plus extra for deep frying

1 tsp cumin seeds

½ tsp turmeric

2.5cm/1in root ginger, ground

2 green chillies, finely chopped

1 tsp amchoor*

Salt to taste

100g/3½oz frozen peas

Method

- Slit each aubergine lengthways and scoop out the flesh.
- Heat the oil. Add the aubergine shells. Deep fry for 2 minutes. Set aside.
- Heat 2 tbsp oil in a saucepan. Add the cumin seeds and turmeric. Let them splutter for 15 seconds. Add the remaining ingredients and the aubergine flesh. Mash lightly and cook on a low heat for 5 minutes.
- Carefully stuff the aubergine shells with this mixture. Grill for 3-4 minutes. Serve hot.

Veggie Bahar

(Vegetables in a Nutty Sauce)

Serves 4

Ingredients

3 tbsp refined vegetable oil

1 large onion, finely chopped

2 large tomatoes, finely chopped

1 tsp ginger paste

1 tsp garlic paste

20 cashew nuts, ground

2 tbsp walnuts, ground

2 tbsp poppy seeds

200g/7oz yoghurt

100g/3½oz frozen mixed vegetables

1 tsp garam masala

Salt to taste

Method

- Heat the oil in a saucepan. Add the onion. Fry on a medium heat till brown. Add the tomatoes, ginger paste, garlic paste, cashew nuts, walnuts and poppy seeds. Fry for 3-4 minutes.
- Add the remaining ingredients. Cook for 7-8 minutes. Serve hot.

Stuffed Vegetables

Serves 4

Ingredients

4 small potatoes

100g/3½oz okra

4 small aubergines

4 tbsp refined vegetable oil

½ tsp mustard seeds

Pinch of asafoetida

For the filling:

250g/9oz besan*

1 tsp ground coriander

1 tsp ground cumin

½ tsp turmeric

1 tsp chilli powder

1 tsp garam masala

Salt to taste

Method

- Mix all the filling ingredients together. Set aside.
- Slit the potatoes, okra and aubergines. Stuff with the filling. Set aside.
- Heat the oil in a saucepan. Add the mustard seeds and asafoetida. Let them splutter for 15 seconds. Add the stuffed vegetables. Cover with a lid and cook on a low heat for 8-10 minutes. Serve hot.

Singhi Aloo

(Drumsticks with Potatoes)

Serves 4

Ingredients

5 tbsp refined vegetable oil

3 small onions, finely chopped

3 green chillies, finely chopped

2 large tomatoes, finely chopped

2 tsp ground coriander

Salt to taste

5 Indian drumsticks*, chopped into 7.5cm/3in pieces

2 large potatoes, chopped

360ml/12fl oz water

Method

- Heat the oil in a saucepan. Add the onions and chillies. Fry them on a low heat for a minute.
- Add the tomatoes, ground coriander and salt. Fry for 2-3 minutes.
- Add the drumsticks, potatoes and water. Mix well. Simmer for 10-12 minutes. Serve hot.

Sindhi Curry

Serves 4

Ingredients

150g/5½oz masoor dhal*

Salt to taste

1 litre/1¾ pints water

4 tomatoes, finely chopped

5 tbsp refined vegetable oil

½ tsp cumin seeds

¼ tsp fenugreek seeds

8 curry leaves

3 green chillies, slit lengthways

¼ tsp asafoetida

4 tbsp besan*

½ tsp chilli powder

½ tsp turmeric

8 okras, slit lengthways

10 French beans, diced

6-7 kokum*

1 large carrot, julienned

1 large potato, diced

Method

- Mix the dhal with the salt and water. Cook this mixture in a saucepan on a medium heat for 45 minutes, stirring occasionally.
- Add the tomatoes and simmer for 7-8 minutes. Set aside.
- Heat the oil in a saucepan. Add the cumin and fenugreek seeds, curry leaves, green chillies and asafoetida. Let them splutter for 30 seconds.
- Add the besan. Fry for a minute, stirring constantly.
- Add the remaining ingredients and the dhal mixture. Mix thoroughly. Simmer for 10 minutes. Serve hot.

Gulnar Kofta

(Paneer Balls In Spinach)

Serves 4

Ingredients

150g/5½oz mixed dry fruits

200g/7oz khoya*

4 large potatoes, boiled and mashed

150g/5½oz paneer*, crumbled

100g/3½oz Cheddar cheese

2 tsp cornflour

Refined vegetable oil for deep frying

2 tsp butter

100g/3½oz spinach, finely chopped

1 tsp single cream

Salt to taste

For the spice mixture:

2 cloves

1cm/½in cinnamon

3 black peppercorns

Method

- Mix the dry fruits with the khoya. Set aside.
- Grind together all the ingredients of the spice mixture. Set aside.
- Mix the potatoes, paneer, cheese and cornflour into a dough. Divide the dough into walnut-sized balls and flatten into discs. Place a portion of the dry fruit-khoya mixture on each disc and seal like a pouch.
- Smooth into walnut-sized balls to make the koftas. Set aside.
- Heat the oil in a frying pan. Add the koftas and deep fry them on a medium heat till they turn golden brown. Drain and set aside in a serving dish.
- Heat the butter in a saucepan. Add the ground spice mixture. Fry for a minute.
- Add the spinach and cook for 2-3 minutes.
- Add the cream and salt. Mix well. Pour this mixture over the koftas. Serve hot.

Paneer Korma

(Rich Paneer Curry)

Serves 4

Ingredients

500g/1lb 2oz paneer*

3 tbsp refined vegetable oil

1 large onion, chopped

2.5cm/1in root ginger, julienned

8 garlic cloves, crushed

2 green chillies, finely chopped

1 large tomato, finely chopped

¼ tsp turmeric

½ tsp ground coriander

½ tsp ground cumin

1 tsp chilli powder

½ tsp garam masala

125g/4½oz yoghurt

Salt to taste

250ml/8fl oz water

2 tbsp coriander leaves, finely chopped

Method

- Grate half of the paneer and chop the remainder into 2.5cm/1in pieces.
- Heat the oil in a frying pan. Add the paneer pieces. Fry them on a medium heat till they turn golden brown. Drain and set aside.
- In the same oil, fry the onion, ginger, garlic and green chillies on a medium heat for 2-3 minutes.
- Add the tomato. Fry for 2 minutes.
- Add the turmeric, ground coriander, ground cumin, chilli powder and garam masala. Mix well. Fry for 2-3 minutes.
- Add the yoghurt, salt and water. Mix well. Simmer for 8-10 minutes.
- Add the fried paneer pieces. Mix well. Simmer for 5 minutes.
- Garnish with the grated paneer and coriander leaves. Serve hot.

Chutney Potatoes

Serves 4

Ingredients

100g/3½oz coriander leaves, finely chopped

4 green chillies

2.5cm/1in root ginger

7 garlic cloves

25g/scant 1oz fresh coconut, grated

1 tbsp lemon juice

1 tsp cumin seeds

1 tsp coriander seeds

½ tsp turmeric

½ tsp chilli powder

Salt to taste

750g/1lb 10oz large potatoes, peeled and chopped into discs

4 tbsp refined vegetable oil

¼ tsp mustard seeds

Method

- Mix the coriander leaves, green chillies, ginger, garlic, coconut, lemon juice, cumin and coriander seeds. Grind this mixture to a fine paste.
- Mix this paste with the turmeric, chilli powder and salt.
- Marinate the potatoes with this mixture for 30 minutes.
- Heat the oil in a saucepan. Add the mustard seeds. Let them splutter for 15 seconds.
- Add the potatoes. Cook them on a low heat for 8-10 minutes, stirring occasionally. Serve hot.

Lobia

(Black Eyed Peas Curry)

Serves 4

Ingredients

400g/14oz black eyed peas, soaked overnight

Pinch of bicarbonate of soda

Salt to taste

1.4 litres/2½ pints water

1 large onion

4 garlic cloves

3 tbsp ghee

2 tsp ground coriander

1 tsp ground cumin

1 tsp amchoor*

½ tsp garam masala

½ tsp chilli powder

¼ tsp turmeric

2 tomatoes, diced

3 green chillies, finely chopped

2 tbsp coriander leaves,

finely chopped

Method

- Mix the black eyed peas with the bicarbonate of soda, salt and 1.2 litres/2 pints of water. Cook this mixture in a saucepan on a medium heat for 45 minutes. Drain and set aside.
- Grind the onion and garlic to a paste.
- Heat the ghee in a saucepan. Add the paste and fry it on a medium heat till it turns brown.
- Add the cooked black eyed peas, the remaining water and all the remaining ingredients, except the coriander leaves. Simmer for 8-10 minutes.
- Garnish with the coriander leaves. Serve hot.

Khatta Meetha Vegetable

(Sweet and Sour Vegetables)

Serves 4

Ingredients

1 tbsp flour

1 tbsp malt vinegar

2 tbsp sugar

50g/1¾oz cabbage, finely chopped into long strips

1 large green pepper, chopped into strips

1 large carrot, chopped into strips

50g/1¾oz French beans, slit and chopped

100g/3½oz baby corn

1 tbsp refined vegetable oil

½ tsp ginger paste

½ tsp garlic paste

2-3 green chillies, finely chopped

4-5 spring onions, finely chopped

125g/4½oz tomato purée

120ml/8fl oz ketchup

Salt to taste

10g/¼oz coriander leaves, finely chopped

Method

- Mix the flour with the vinegar and sugar. Set aside.
- Mix together the cabbage, green pepper, carrot, French beans and baby corn. Steam (see cooking techniques) this mixture in a steamer for 10 minutes. Set aside.
- Heat the oil in a saucepan. Add the ginger paste, garlic paste and chillies. Fry for 30 seconds.
- Add the spring onions. Fry for 1-2 minutes.
- Add the steamed vegetables and the tomato purée, ketchup and salt. Cook on a low heat for 5-6 minutes.
- Add the flour paste. Cook for 3-4 minutes.
- Garnish with the coriander leaves. Serve hot.

Dahiwale Chhole

(Chickpea in Yoghurt Sauce)

Serves 4

Ingredients

500g/1lb 2oz chickpeas, soaked overnight

Pinch of bicarbonate of soda

Salt to taste

1 litre/1¾ pints water

3 tbsp ghee

2 large onions, grated

1 tsp ginger, grated

150g/5½oz yoghurt

1 tsp garam masala

1 tsp ground cumin, dry roasted (see cooking techniques)

½ tsp chilli powder

¼ tsp turmeric

1 tsp amchoor*

½ tbsp cashew nuts

½ tbsp raisins

Method

- Mix the chickpeas with the bicarbonate of soda, salt and water. Cook this mixture in a saucepan on a medium heat for 45 minutes. Drain and set aside.
- Heat the ghee in a saucepan. Add the onions and ginger. Fry them on a medium heat till the onions are translucent.
- Add the chickpeas and the remaining ingredients, except the cashew nuts and raisins. Mix well. Cook on a low heat for 7-8 minutes.
- Garnish with the cashew nuts and raisins. Serve hot.

Teekha Papad Bhaji*

(Spicy Poppadam Dish)

Serves 4

Ingredients

1 tbsp refined vegetable oil

¼ tsp mustard seeds

¼ tsp cumin seeds

¼ tsp fenugreek seeds

2 tsp ground coriander

3 tsp sugar

Salt to taste

250ml/8fl oz water

6 poppadams, broken into bits

1 tbsp coriander leaves, chopped

Method

- Heat the oil in a saucepan. Add the mustard, cumin and fenugreek seeds, ground coriander, sugar and salt. Let them splutter for 30 seconds. Add the water and simmer for 3-4 minutes.
- Add the poppadam pieces. Simmer for 5-7 minutes. Garnish with the coriander leaves. Serve hot.

www.ingramcontent.com/pod-product-compliance
Lightning Source LLC
Chambersburg PA
CBHW071823080526
44589CB00012B/893